# 100 CASES
## in Obstetrics and Gynaecology

# 100 CASES
## in Obstetrics and Gynaecology

Cecilia Bottomley MB BChir MRCOG
Clinical Lecturer in Obstetrics and Gynaecology, St George's, University of London, UK

Janice Rymer MD FRCOG FRANZCOG FHEA
Professor of Obstetrics and Gynaecology, King's College London School of Medicine
at Guy's, King's and St Thomas' Hospitals, London, UK

100 Cases Series Editor:
P John Rees MD FRCP
Dean of Medical Undergraduate Education, King's College London School
of Medicine at Guy's, King's and St Thomas' Hospitals, London, UK

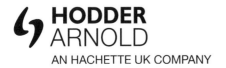

**HODDER**
ARNOLD
AN HACHETTE UK COMPANY

First published in Great Britain in 2008 by
Hodder Arnold, an imprint of Hodder Education, an Hachette UK Company
338 Euston Road, London NW1 3BH

http://www.hoddereducation.com

Whilst the advice and information in this book are believed to be true and accurate at the date
of going to press, neither the author[s] nor the publisher can accept any legal responsibility or
liability for any errors or omissions that may be made. In particular, (but without limiting the
generality of the preceding disclaimer) every effort has been made to check drug dosages;
however it is still possible that errors have been missed. Furthermore, dosage schedules are
constantly being revised and new side-effects recognized. For these reasons the reader is
strongly urged to consult the drug companies' printed instructions before administering any of
the drugs recommended in this book.

*British Library Cataloguing in Publication Data*
A catalogue record for this book is available from the British Library

*Library of Congress Cataloging-in-Publication Data*
A catalog record for this book is available from the Library of Congress

ISBN          978 0 340 94744 9

5  6  7  8  9  10

| Commissioning Editor: | Sara Purdy |
| Project Editor: | Jane Tod |
| Production Controller: | Andre Sim |
| Cover Design: | Laura DeGrasse |
| Indexer: | Indexing Specialists (UK) Ltd |

Typeset in 10/12 RotisSerif by Charon Tec Ltd (A MacMillan Company), Chennai, India
www.charontec.com
Printed and bound in India

What do you think about this book? Or any other Hodder Arnold title?
Please visit our website: www.hoddereducation.com

# CONTENTS

# PREFACE

Learning in medicine has gradually moved away from an apprentice system to a more structured course format. Advances have been made with the use of simulated cases, problem-based learning and electronic learning resources; however, this has led to a separation of the learning environment from the clinical art of real medicine.

This book aims to redress the balance with entirely clinical cases, highlighting the history and examination features with salient investigations. This allows the reader to place themselves in the position of the practising doctor encountering these scenarios in the everyday clinical setting.

Obstetrics and gynaecology involves the same clinical reasoning as other specialties covered in this series, but several points should be highlighted. First most patients seen in obstetrics and gynaecology are generally fit and healthy. As such they will withstand cardiovascular insults such as haemorrhage very effectively by increasing cardiac output. Signs of tachycardia and hypovolaemia may be late and signify severe compromise. Second, there are many physiological changes in pregnancy and normal ranges therefore alter. Where indicated, normal values for pregnant and non-pregnant women have been included. Finally, many abnormalities in obstetrics and gynaecology are picked up during 'routine' care. This book therefore differs from those of Clinical Medicine and Surgery in that women do not always 'present' with a problem, but one may be detected through, for example, routine antenatal care or during a cervical smear investigation.

The cases are grouped into broad categories with random ordering of cases within each category to mimic the way cases present in clinical practice.

We have written this book with both clinicians and medical students in mind, with cases varying in complexity, to reinforce common or important subject areas. We hope they will stimulate and challenge as well as build confidence for those working in or learning obstetrics and gynaecology.

Cecilia Bottomley
Janice Rymer
January 2008

# ACKNOWLEDGEMENTS

The authors would like to thank the following people for their help with illustrations and useful suggestions for cases: Dr Anna Belli, Mr Tom Bourne, Miss Jan Grace, Mr Kevin Hayes, Dr Emma Kirk, Miss Gini Lowe, Dr Jasper Verguts and Dr Miles Walkden.

# ABBREVIATIONS

| | |
|---|---|
| AFP | alpha-fetoprotein |
| APH | antepartum haemorrhage |
| APTT | activated partial thromboplastin time |
| ARM | artificial rupture of membranes |
| BMI | body mass index |
| BV | bacterial vaginosis |
| CIN | cervical intraepithelial neoplasia |
| COCP | combined oral contraceptive pill |
| CT | computerized tomography |
| CTG | cardiotocograph |
| CTPA | computerized tomography pulmonary angiogram |
| CVS | chorionic villous sampling |
| DCDA | dichorionic diamniotic |
| DIC | disseminated intravascular coagulopathy |
| DUB | dysfunctional uterine bleeding |
| EAS | external anal sphincter |
| ECG | electrocardiogram |
| EIA | enzyme immunoassay |
| ERPC | evacuation of retained products of conception |
| FBS | fetal blood sampling |
| FSH | follicle-stimulating hormone |
| FTA-abs | treponemal antibody-absorbed (test) |
| GBS | group B streptococcus |
| GDM | gestational diabetes mellitus |
| GP | general practitioner |
| Hb | haemoglobin |
| HCG | human chorionic gonadotrophin |
| HELLP | haemolysis, elevated liver enzymes and low platelets |
| HIV | human immunodeficiency virus |
| HRT | hormone replacement therapy |
| IAS | internal anal sphincter |
| Ig | immunoglobulin |
| INR | international normalized ratio |
| IUCD | intrauterine contraceptive device |
| IUS | intrauterine system |
| IVF | in vitro fertilization |
| LLETZ | large-loop excision of the transformation zone |
| LH | luteinizing hormone |
| LMP | last menstrual period date |
| MCH | mean cell haemoglobin |
| MoM | multiples of the median |
| MRI | magnetic resonance imaging |

| NT | nuchal translucency |
| OAB | overactive bladder syndrome |
| OC | obstetric cholestasis |
| PCA | patient-controlled analgesia |
| PCOS | polycystic ovarian syndrome |
| PE | pulmonary embolism |
| PIH | pregnancy-induced hypertension |
| PMB | postmenopausal bleeding |
| PMS | premenstrual syndrome |
| POP | progesterone only pill |
| PPH | postpartum haemorrhage |
| PUL | pregnancy of unknown location |
| RDS | respiratory distress syndrome |
| SLE | systemic lupus erythematosus |
| SPD | symphysiopelvic dysfunction |
| STI | sexually transmitted infection |
| TCRF | transcervical resection of a fibroid |
| TEDS | thromboembolic stockings |
| TIBC | total iron-binding capacity |
| TPN | total parenteral nutrition |
| TSH | thyroid-stimulating hormone |
| $T_3$ | tri-iodothyronine |
| $T_4$ | thyroxine |
| UTI | urinary tract infection |
| VBAC | vaginal birth after Caesarean |
| VDRL | venereal disease research laboratory (test) |
| VTE | venous thromboembolism |
| WHO | World Health Organization |

# GENERAL GYNAECOLOGY

## CASE 1: INTERMENSTRUAL BLEEDING

### History

A 48-year-old woman presents with intermenstrual bleeding for 2 months. Episodes of bleeding occur any time in the cycle. This is usually fresh red blood and much lighter than a normal period. It can last for 1–6 days. There is no associated pain. She has no hot flushes or night sweats. She is sexually active and has not noticed vaginal dryness.

She has three children and has used the progesterone only pill for contraception for 5 years.

Her last smear test was 2 years ago and all smears have been normal. She takes no medication and has no other relevant medical history.

### Examination

The abdomen is unremarkable. Speculum examination shows a slightly atrophic-looking vagina and cervix but there are no apparent cervical lesions and there is no current bleeding.

On bimanual examination the uterus is non-tender and of normal size, axial and mobile. There are no adnexal masses.

| INVESTIGATIONS | | Normal range |
| --- | --- | --- |
| Haemoglobin | 12.7 g/dL | 11.7–15.7g/dL |
| White cell count | $4.5 \times 10^9$/L | $3.5–11 \times 10^9$/L |
| Platelets | $401 \times 10^9$/L | $150–440 \times 10^9$/L |

Transvaginal ultrasound scan and hydrosonography is shown in Fig. 1.1.

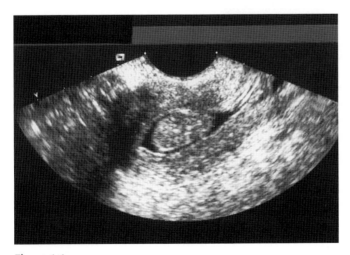

Figure 1.1

### Questions
- What is the diagnosis and differential diagnosis?
- How would you further investigate and manage this woman?

# ANSWER 1

The diagnosis is of an endometrial polyp, as shown by the hydrosonography image (Fig. 1.1). These can occur in women of any age although they are more common in older women and may be asymptomatic or cause irregular bleeding or discharge. The aetiology is uncertain and the vast majority are benign. In this specific case all the differential diagnoses are effectively excluded by the history and examination.

> **!  Differential diagnosis for intermenstrual bleeding**
>
> - Cervical malignancy
> - Cervical ectropion
> - Endocervical polyp
> - Atrophic vaginitis
> - Pregnancy
> - Irregular bleeding related to the contraceptive pill

## Management

Any woman should be investigated if bleeding occurs between periods. In women over the age of 40 years, serious pathology, in particular endometrial carcinoma, should be excluded.

The polyp needs to be removed for two reasons:

1  to eliminate the cause of the bleeding
2  to obtain a histological report to ensure that it is not malignant.

Management involves outpatient or day case hysteroscopy, and resection of the polyp under direct vision using a diathermy loop or other resection technique (Fig. 1.2). This allows certainty that the polyp had been completely excised and also allows full inspection of the rest of the cavity to check for any other lesions or suspicious areas. In some settings, where hysteroscopic facilities are not available, a dilatation and curettage may be carried out with blind avulsion of the polyp with polyp forceps. This was the standard management in the past but is not the gold standard now, for the reasons explained.

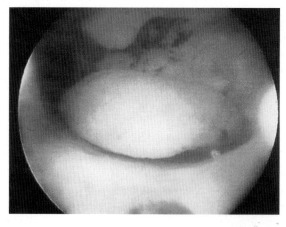

**Figure 1.2** Hysteroscopic appearance of endometrial polyp prior to resection. See Plate 1 for colour image.

> **🔑  KEY POINTS**
>
> - Any woman over the age of 40 years should be investigated if bleeding occurs between the periods, to exclude serious pathology, in particular endometrial carcinoma.
> - Hysteroscopy and dilatation and curettage is rarely indicated for women under the age of 40 years.

# CASE 2: INFERTILITY

### History

A 31-year-old woman has been trying to conceive for nearly 3 years without success. Her last period started 7 months ago and she has been having periods sporadically for about 5 years. She bleeds for 2–7 days and the periods occur with an interval of 2–9 months. There is no dysmenorrhoea but occasionally the bleeding is heavy.

She was pregnant once before at the age of 19 years and had a termination of pregnancy. She had a laparoscopy several years ago for pelvic pain, which showed a normal pelvis.

Cervical smears have always been normal and there is no history of sexually transmitted infection.

The woman was diagnosed with irritable bowel syndrome when she was 25, after thorough investigation for other bowel conditions. She currently uses metoclopramide to increase gut motility, and antispasmodics.

Her partner is fit and well, and has two children by a previous relationship. Neither partner drinks alcohol or smokes.

| INVESTIGATIONS | | |
|---|---|---|
| | | *Normal* |
| Follicle-stimulating hormone | 3.1 IU/L | Day 2–5 |
| | | 1–11 IU/L |
| Luteinizing hormone | 2.9 IU/L | Day 2–5 |
| | | 0.5–14.5 IU/L |
| Day 21 progesterone | 12 nmol/L | |
| Prolactin | 1274 mu/L | 90–520 mu/L |
| Testosterone | 1.4 nmol/L | 0.8–3.1 nmol/L |
| Thyroid-stimulating hormone | 4.1 mu/L | 0.5–7 mu/L |
| Free thyroxine | 17 pmol/L | 11–23 pmol/L |

### Questions
- What is the diagnosis and its aetiology?
- How would you further investigate and manage this couple?

# ANSWER 2

The infertility is secondary to anovulation as shown by the day 21 progesterone (>30 nmol/L suggests ovulation has occurred). Normal testosterone and gonadotrophins and high prolactin suggest the likely case of anovulation is hyperprolactinaemia. Hyperprolactinaemia may be physiological in breast-feeding, pregnancy and stress. The commonest causes of pathological hyperprolactinaemia are tumours and idiopathic hypersecretion, but it may also be due to drugs, hypothyroidism, ectopic prolactin secretion or chronic renal failure. In this case the metoclopramide is the cause, as it is a dopamine antagonist (dopamine usually acts via the hypothalamus to cause inhibition of prolactin secretion, and if this is interrupted, prolactin is excreted to excess). Galactorrhoea is not a common symptom of hyperprolactinaemia, occurring in less than half of affected women.

---

**!**   **Drugs associated with hyperprolactinaemia (due to dopamine antagonist effects)**

- Metoclopramide
- Phenothiazines (e.g. chlorpromazine, prochlorperazine, thioridazine)
- Reserpine
- Methyldopa
- Omeprazole, ranitidine, bendrofluazide (rare associations)

---

The metoclopramide should be stopped and the woman reviewed after 4–6 weeks to ensure that the periods have restarted and that the prolactin level has returned to normal. If this does not occur, then further investigation is needed to exclude other causes of hyperprolactinaemia such as a pituitary micro- or macro-adenoma. It would be advisable to repeat the day 21 progesterone level to confirm ovulatory cycles. The woman should have her rubella immunity checked and should be advised to take preconceptual folic acid until 12 weeks of pregnancy.

If the woman fails to conceive then a full fertility investigation should be planned with semen analysis and tubal patency testing (hysterosalpingogram or laparoscopy and dye test).

---

   **KEY POINTS**

- A full drug history should be elicited in women with amenorrhoea or infertility.
- Galactorrhoea occurs in less than half of women with hyperprolactinaemia.
- Day 21 progesterone over 30 nmol/L is suggestive of ovulation.

---

# CASE 3: AMENORRHOEA

## History

A 32-year-old woman complains that she has not had a period for 3 months. Four home pregnancy tests have all been negative. She started her periods at the age of 15 years and until 30 years she had a normal 27-day cycle. She had one daughter by normal delivery 2 years ago, following which she breast-fed for 6 months. After that she had normal cycles again for several months and then her periods stopped abruptly. She was using the progesterone only pill for contraception while she was breast-feeding and stopped 6 months ago as she is keen to have another child. She reports symptoms of dryness during intercourse and has experienced sweating episodes at night as well as episodes of feeling extremely hot at any time of day. There is no relevant gynaecological history. The only medical history of note is that she has been hypothyroid for 10 years and takes thyroxine 100 μg per day. She does not take any alcohol, smoke or use recreational drugs.

## Examination

Examination findings are unremarkable

### INVESTIGATIONS

|  |  | Normal range |
|---|---|---|
| Haemoglobin | 12.2 g/dL | 11.7–15.7 g/dL |
| White cell count | 5.1 × 10⁹/L | 3.5–11 × 10⁹/L |
| Platelets | 203 × 10⁹/L | 150–440 × 10⁹/L |
| Thyroid-stimulating hormone | 3.6 mu/L | 0.5–7 mu/L |
| Free thyroxine | 28 pmol/L | 11–23 pmol/L |
| Follicle-stimulating hormone | 45 IU/L | Day 2–5 1–11 IU/L |
| Luteinizing hormone | 30 IU/L | Day 2–5 0.5–14.5 IU/L |
| Prolactin | 401 mu/L | 90–520 mu/L |
| Oestradiol | 87 pmol/L | Day 2–5 70–510 pmol/L |
| Testosterone | 2.3 nmol/L | 0.8–3.1 nmol/L |

## Questions

- What is the diagnosis?
- What further investigations should be performed?
- What are the important points in the management of this woman?

# ANSWER 3

This woman has symptoms of amenorrhoea as well as hypo-oestrogenic vasomotor symptoms and vaginal dryness. The diagnosis is of premature menopause, confirmed by the very high gonadotrophin levels. High levels occur because the ovary is resistant to the effects of gonadotrophins, and negative feedback to the hypothalamus and pituitary causes increasing secretion to try and stimulate the ovary. Sheehan's syndrome (pituitary necrosis after postpartum haemorrhage) would also cause amenorrhoea but would have inhibited breast-feeding and all menstruation since delivery.

Premature menopause (before the age of 40 years) occurs in 1 per cent of women and has significant physical and psychological consequences. It may be idiopathic but a familial tendency is common. In some cases it is an autoimmune condition (associated with hypothyroidism in this case). Disorders of the X chromosome can also be associated.

> **! Effects of premature menopause**
>
> - *Hypo-oestrogenic effects*:
>   - vaginal dryness
>   - vasomotor symptoms (hot flushes, night sweats)
>   - osteoporosis
>   - increased cardiovascular risk
> - *Psychological and social effects*:
>   - infertility
>   - feeling of inadequacy as a woman
>   - feelings of premature ageing and need to take hormone-replacement therapy (HRT)
>   - impact on relationships

## Further investigations

Repeat gonadotrophin level is required to confirm the result and exclude a midcycle gonadotrophin surge or fluctuating gonadotrophins. Bone scan is necessary for baseline bone density and to help in monitoring the effects of hormone replacement. Chromosomal analysis identifies the rare cases of premature menopause due to fragile X syndrome or Turner's syndrome mosaicism.

## Management

Osteoporosis may be prevented with oestrogen replacement, with progesterone protection of the uterus. Traditional HRT preparations or the combined oral contraceptive pill are effective, the latter making women feel more 'normal', with a monthly withdrawal bleed and a 'young person's' medication.

Her options are adoption, accepting childlessness and in vitro fertilization (IVF) with donor oocytes.

Occasionally premature menopause is a fluctuating condition (resistant ovary syndrome) whereby the ovaries may function intermittently. Contraception should therefore be used if it would be undesirable to become pregnant.

Patient support organizations are a good source for women experiencing such an unexpected and stigmatizing diagnosis.

>  **KEY POINTS**
>
> - Premature menopause (<40 years) occurs in 1 per cent of women.
> - Oestrogen replacement is essential for bone and cardiovascular protection.
> - It may be possible to conceive with IVF using donor oocytes.

## CASE 4: INFERTILITY

### History

A 29-year-old woman and her partner are seen in the gynaecology outpatient clinic with primary infertility. They stopped using condoms 2 years ago and have had regular intercourse since then. The partner has no previous medical history of note. He drinks approximately 8 units of alcohol per week and does not smoke. He works as a manager in a hotel.

The woman also has no specific previous medical history except for an appendectomy aged 12 years. Her periods occur every 31 to 46 days and can be heavy at times but not painful. There is no intermenstrual or postcoital bleeding. She has always had normal smears and has never had any sexually transmitted infections. She takes no medications, drinks approximately 6 units of alcohol per week and does not smoke.

### Examination

On examination her body mass index (BMI) is $29 \, \text{kg/m}^2$. She has slight acne on her face and her chest.

There are no abdominal scars and the abdomen is non-tender with no masses palpable. Speculum and bimanual examination are normal.

| INVESTIGATIONS | | |
|---|---|---|
| | | *Normal* |
| Day 3 luteinizing hormone (LH) | 6.2 IU/L | Day 2–5 0.5–14.5 IU/L |
| Day 3 follicle-stimulating hormone | 3.1 IU/L | Day 2–5 1–11 IU/L |
| Testosterone | 4.1 nmol/L | 0.8–3.1 nmol/L |
| Day 21 progesterone | 15 nmol/L | |

A transvaginal ultrasound scan is shown in Fig. 4.1.

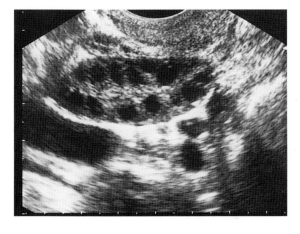

Figure 4.1 Transvaginal ultrasound scan.

### Questions
- What is the diagnosis?
- How would you further investigate and manage this woman?

# ANSWER 4

The diagnosis is of anovulatory infertility due to polycystic ovarian syndrome (PCOS). Anovulation is shown by the progesterone level below 30 nmol/L, and PCOS is suggested by several features including increased BMI, acne, oligomenorrhoea, polycystic ovaries on transvaginal ultrasound examination, increased androgen levels and increased LH.

'Polycystic ovaries' (a morphological description of enlarged ovaries with an increased number of follicles and dense stroma) is present in up to 25 per cent of normal women. The diagnosis of PCOS is made on any combination of characteristic clinical, biochemical and ultrasound features.

PCOS is one of the commonest causes of infertility. However, up to 30 per cent of sub-fertile couples have a multifactorial cause for their problem. Hence complete investigation of both partners is essential prior to treating the PCOS. This includes:

- semen analysis
- tubal patency test (hysterosalpingogram is usually sufficient)
- laparoscopy and dye test if pelvic inflammatory disease, adhesions or endometriosis are suggested from the history.

Testing for rubella is also necessary, as is a recommendation to take folic acid if this is not already taken. Other general advice includes minimizing alcohol intake, avoiding smoking and ensuring regular intercourse (preferably 2–3 times per week). The woman should aim to reduce weight as this commonly induces ovulation in high-BMI women with PCOS.

### Treatment of anovulation

Clomifene citrate is the main treatment to induce ovulation. The woman should be given 50 mg to take on day 2–6 of the menstrual cycle, with day 21 progesterone checked to confirm ovulation. If ovulation occurs, then the clomifene is continued for up to six cycles unless pregnancy occurs. If ovulation is not confirmed then the dose is increased to 100 mg.

It is not recommended to take clomifene for more than 6 months, due to a theoretical increased risk of ovarian carcinoma. If clomifene fails, then further ovulation induction agents and IVF need to be considered.

---

 **KEY POINTS**

- Irregular periods are commonly due to polycystic ovarian syndrome.
- The syndrome is diagnosed on a combination of clinical, biochemical and ultrasound features.
- Many cases of subfertility are multifactorial or involve both partners, so full investigation of both is important prior to treatment.

# CASE 5: INFERTILITY

## History

A 37-year-old woman is seen in the clinic because of infertility. She is gravida 3 para 1 having had a daughter 13 years ago and a miscarriage 2 years later. She separated from her former husband and has now married again and is keen to conceive, especially as her new partner has no children.

Her last period started 45 days ago. She says that her periods are sometimes regular but at other times she has missed a period for up to 3 months. The bleeding is moderate and lasts up to 4 days. There is no history of pelvic pain or dyspareunia, and no irregular bleeding or discharge. Alcohol intake is minimal and she does not smoke or take other drugs. There is no medical history of note and she takes no regular medication.

Her partner is 34 years old and is also fit and healthy with no significant history of ill-health or medications.

## Examination

There are no abnormal features on examination of either partner.

---

### INVESTIGATIONS (DURING THE NEXT MENSTRUAL CYCLE)

|  |  | *Normal* |
|---|---|---|
| Day 3 follicle-stimulating hormone (FSH) | 11.1 IU/L | Day 2–5 1–11 IU/L |
| Day 3 luteinizing hormone | 6.8 IU/L | Day 2–5 0.5–14.5 IU/L |
| Prolactin | 305 mu/L | 90–520 mu/L |
| Testosterone | 1.3 nmol/L | 0.8–3.1 nmol/L |
| Day 21 progesterone | 23 nmol/L | |

*Semen analysis report*: normal volume, count, normal forms and motility.

*Hysterosalpingogram report*: the uterine cavity is of normal shape with a smooth regular outline. Contrast medium is seen to fill both uterine tubes symmetrically and free spill of dye is confirmed bilaterally.

*Transvaginal ultrasound scan report*: the uterus is anteverted with no congenital abnormalities, uterine fibroids or polyps visualized. Both ovaries are of normal morphology, volume and mobility. No follicles are noted.

---

## Questions

- What is the cause of the infertility?
- What are the further investigation and management options?

# ANSWER 5

Women with irregular periods often do not ovulate. Anovulation in this case is confirmed by the low day 21 progesterone level. The commonest cause of anovulation is polycystic ovaries, but in this case the ovaries show normal morphology and the androgen levels are normal.

The noticeable abnormality is the high FSH level and the fact that no follicles are visualized at ultrasound scan. This is suggestive of anovulation from premature failure of ovarian function. The woman is not menopausal because she still has periods although irregular, and the FSH is only marginally raised. However it is known that FSH levels above 10 IU/L are associated with a poor prognosis for conception using the woman's own ova.

## Further investigation.

The FSH should be repeated, as it is possible that this could be a sporadic result or poorly timed sample, and therefore confirmation is needed before continuing on to treatment.

## Management

As there is such a poor prognosis for conception either naturally or with in vitro fertilization using the woman's own ova, she should be counselled about assisted conception using donor eggs. Donated oocytes are fertilized with the partner's sperm and then implanted into the uterus. The woman needs appropriate luteal phase support, most commonly with progesterone pessaries.

---

**!**  **Counselling issues for this couple**

- *Psychological*:
    - the woman may feel that her ovaries are 'ageing' prematurely and this may have an affect on her self-esteem and sexuality
    - the stress associated with assisted conception is significant and many couples find that this in itself puts a large burden on their relationship.
- *Funding*: public funding may not be available as the woman already has one child.
- *Consideration of alternative options*: adoption, surrogacy and accepting childlessness should be explored with the couple.

---

  **KEY POINTS**

- FSH above 10 IU/L is associated with poor prognosis for fertility.
- Infertile couples should be encouraged to explore all options, including accepting childlessness and adoption as well as assisted conception techniques.

# CASE 6: SHORTNESS OF BREATH AND ABDOMINAL PAIN

## History

A 72-year-old woman has been admitted with shortness of breath. On further questioning she says she has been unwell for about 8 weeks. She has decreased appetite and nausea when she eats. She has lost weight but her abdomen feels swollen. She has generalized dull abdominal pain and constipation, which is unusual for her. There are no urinary symptoms.

She has always been healthy with no previous hospital admissions. She is a widow and did not have any children. Her periods stopped at 52 years and she has had no post-menopausal bleeding. She has never taken hormone-replacement therapy.

## Examination

She appears pale and breathless on talking. Chest expansion is reduced on the right side, with dullness to percussion and decreased air entry at the right base. The abdomen is generally distended with shifting dullness. There is a mass arising from the pelvis. Speculum examination is normal, but on bimanual palpation there is a fixed left iliac fossa mass of about 10 cm diameter.

| INVESTIGATIONS | | |
|---|---|---|
| | | Normal |
| Haemoglobin | 9.2 g/dL | 11.7–15.7 g/dL |
| Mean cell volume | 82 fL | 80–99 fL |
| White cell count | $4.1 \times 10^9$/L | $3.5–11 \times 10^9$/L |
| Platelets | $197 \times 10^9$/L | $150–440 \times 10^9$/L |
| Sodium | 135 mmol/L | 135–145 mmol/L |
| Potassium | 4.0 mmol/L | 3.5–5 mmol/L |
| Urea | 5.1 mmol/L | 2.5–6.7 mmol/L |
| Creatinine | 89 μmol/L | 70–120 μmol/L |
| Alanine transaminase | 18 IU/L | 5–35 IU/L |
| Aspartate transaminase | 17 IU/L | 5–35 IU/L |
| Alkaline phosphatase | 78 IU/L | 30–300 IU/L |
| Bilirubin | 12 μmol/L | 3–17 μmol/L |
| Albumin | 30 g/L | 35–50 g/L |
| CA-125 | 118 ku/L | <30 ku/L |

Chest X-ray and abdominal computerized tomography (CT) scan are shown in Figs 6.1 and 6.2 respectively.

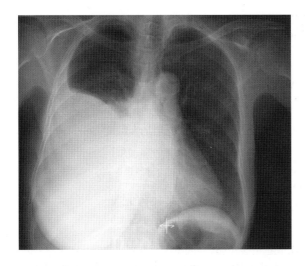

**Figure 6.1** Chest X-ray.

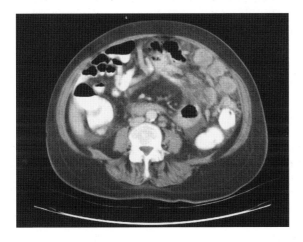

**Figure 6.2** Abdominal CT scan.

## Questions

- What is the likely diagnosis?
- How should this woman be further investigated?
- If the diagnosis is confirmed how should she be managed?

# ANSWER 6

The history and examination are suggestive of a right pleural effusion and ascites. The presence of a pelvic mass would suggest that this is due to an ovarian or bowel problem. The chest X-ray confirms the effusion, and the CT shows a left-sided pelvic tumour and ascites. There are also solid areas in the anterior abdominal wall that represent omental infiltration by the tumour.

CA-125 is a non-specific marker for ovarian carcinoma. The diagnosis is therefore likely to be that of ovarian cancer which commonly presents with systemic symptoms when metastatic disease is already evident.

## Confirmation of the diagnosis and management

The surgical aphorism 'there is no diagnosis without a surgical diagnosis' means that tissue needs to be obtained to confirm the diagnosis. Laparotomy should be performed with three objectives:

1 obtaining tissue for diagnosis
2 staging the disease according to the extent of tissue involvement
3 primary debulking – to perform a total abdominal hysterectomy and bilateral salpingoophorectomy and to reduce all abdominal tumour deposits to a volume of less than 2 cm. This allows optimal effect of chemotherapy following surgery. Lymph node dissection and omental resection are usually part of the procedure.

Prior to any treatment this woman also needs drainage of her pleural effusion for symptomatic relief and optimization for anaesthetic.

The prognosis for ovarian cancer is poor, as most women present at stage 3 or 4.

---

 **KEY POINTS**

- CA-125 is a non-specific marker for ovarian cancer.
- Ovarian cancer commonly presents late (stage 3/4) and prognosis is poor.
- Staging and primary treatment is by laparotomy, total abdominal hysterectomy, bilateral salpingoophorectomy and debulking.
- Chemotherapy is often effective adjuvant therapy.

## CASE 7: ABDOMINAL SWELLING

### History

A 36-year-old African-Caribbean woman has noticed abdominal swelling for 10 months. She has to wear larger clothes and people have asked her if she is pregnant, which she finds distressing having been trying to conceive. She has no abdominal pain and her bowel habit is normal. She feels nauseated when she eats large amounts. She has urinary frequency but no dysuria or haematuria.

Her periods are regular, every 27 days, and have always been heavy, with clots and flooding on the second and third days. She has never received any treatment for her heavy periods.

She has been with her partner for 7 years and despite not using contraception she has never been pregnant.

### Examination

The woman has a very distended abdomen. A smooth firm mass is palpable extending from the symphysis pubis to midway between the umbilicus and the xiphisternum (equivalent to a 32-week size pregnancy). It is non-tender and mobile. It is not fluctuant and it is not possible to palpate beneath the mass. On speculum examination it is not possible to visualize the cervix. Bimanual examination reveals a non-tender firm mass occupying the pelvis.

---

🔍 **INVESTIGATIONS**

|                    |                      | Normal                      |
|--------------------|----------------------|-----------------------------|
| Haemoglobin        | 6.3 g/dL             | 11.7–15.7 g/dL              |
| Mean cell volume   | 68 fL                | 80–99 fL                    |
| White cell count   | $4.9 \times 10^9$/L  | $3.5–11 \times 10^9$/L      |
| Platelets          | $267 \times 10^9$/L  | $150–440 \times 10^9$/L     |

Magnetic resonance images (MRI) of the abdomen and pelvis are shown in Figs 7.1 and 7.2.

---

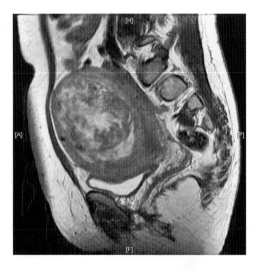

**Figure 7.1** MRI of the abdomen and pelvis.

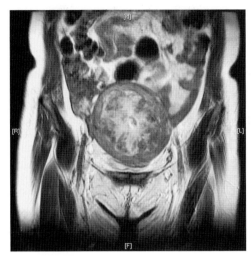

Figure 7.2 MRI of the abdomen and pelvis.

## Questions
- What is the diagnosis?
- How would you further investigate and manage this woman?

# ANSWER 7

The woman has a large uterine fibroid (leiomyoma). This is causing menorrhagia and hence the microcytic anaemia from iron deficiency. It is also likely that the fibroid is accounting for her infertility history, although this warrants investigation as a separate problem.

Fibroids are benign tumours of the myometrium which may be extrinsic (subserous) as in this case. Alternatively they may be intramural or submucosal (projecting into the endometrial cavity).

---

 **Typical presentations of fibroids**

- Menorrhagia
- Abdominal mass
- Pressure effect from pressure on the bladder, stomach or bowel
- Infertility

---

Fibroids are not typically painful unless they undergo degeneration, usually in pregnancy.

African-Caribbean women tend to develop fibroids more commonly than other ethnic groups.

### Further investigation
Ferritin and folate levels should be checked to confirm the iron-deficiency status. It is also advisable to arrange renal function tests and a renal tract ultrasound, as very large fibroids can cause ureteric obstruction and hydronephrosis, which would need urgent treatment.

### Management
The woman should be treated for her anaemia with ferrous sulphate. The menorrhagia can be reduced with tranexamic acid during menstruation. Gonadotrophin-releasing hormone analogues temporarily shrink fibroids and cause amenorrhoea to allow correction of iron deficiency. Definitive treatment for fibroids is traditionally by hysterectomy or myomectomy. Myomectomy is favourable for this woman who is keen to have a family, so conservation of the uterus is essential. Uterine artery embolization also causes fibroid degeneration by interruption of the blood supply. However research into long-term safety and potential effects on uterine function during pregnancy are not clear, and this option is currently advised in the context of a research setting only.

---

 **KEY POINTS**

- Fibroids may be small and incidental or occupy most of the abdomen.
- Anaemia should be suspected in any women with menorrhagia.
- Treatment of fibroids depends on the presence of symptoms and the necessity to preserve fertility.
- The optimal operative approach depends on the size and location of the fibroids.

---

# CASE 8: ABNORMAL CERVICAL SMEAR

### History

A 28-year-old woman attends the colposcopy clinic after an abnormal smear test. She is very anxious as she thinks that she might have cervical cancer. The smear is reported as 'severe dyskaryosis'. She had a previous normal result at age 25 years. She has not had any postcoital or intermenstrual bleeding.

Her first sexual relationship started at the age of 14 years and she has had several partners since then. She lives with her current partner who she has been with for 3 years. She was diagnosed with genital herpes several years ago but has not had any attacks for at least 3 years. She smokes 15–20 cigarettes per day and drinks only at the weekends.

She has an intrauterine contraceptive device in situ.

### Examination

The cervix is macroscopically normal. At colposcopy, acetic acid is applied and an irregular white area is apparent to the left of the os. Lugol's iodine is applied and the same area stains pale while the rest of the cervix stains dark brown. A biopsy is taken

---

 **INVESTIGATIONS**

*Cervical biopsy report*: the sample received measures 4 mm × 2 mm and contains enlarged cells with irregular nuclei consistent with CIN3.

---

### Questions
• How should this patient be managed?

# ANSWER 8

The colposcopy findings show an abnormal area on the left of the cervix. The abnormal tissue stains white with acetic acid because abnormal cells have high-density nuclei which take up the acetic acid more than normal cells. In contrast, abnormal cells have lower glycogen content than normal cells and stain less well, remaining pale when iodine is applied.

The diagnosis is of CIN3 (cervical intraepithelial neoplasia). This is a tissue diagnosis as opposed to dyskaryosis which is an observation of cells from a smear. The degree of dyskaryosis and CIN often correlate, but a dyskaryosis report is not a diagnosis.

## Management

CIN needs to be treated to prevent progression over several years to cervical carcinoma. The commonest treatment is large-loop excision of the transformation zone (LLETZ) – removal of abnormal cervical tissue with a diathermy loop. Most women tolerate this under local anaesthetic. The LLETZ sample needs to be examined histologically both to confirm removal of all the abnormal tissue, and to ensure that there is not a focus of carcinoma within the sample.

Follow-up smear should be performed in 6 months, and thereafter yearly smears for 10 years.

---

**!  Advice after LLETZ procedure**

- The patient may have light bleeding for several days.
- If heavy bleeding occurs she should return as secondary infection may occur and need treatment.
- She should avoid sexual intercourse and tampon use for 4 weeks, to allow healing of the cervix.
- Fertility is generally unaffected by the procedure, though cervical stenosis leading to infertility has been reported, and mid-trimester loss from cervical weakness is rare.

---

**KEY POINTS**

- Dyskariosis refers to abnormality from a smear.
- Dysplasia or cervical intraepithelial neoplasia are histological terms from a biopsy sample.
- CIN should be treated to prevent long-term progression to cervical carcinoma.
- LLETZ is the usual treatment for CIN, with yearly follow-up for 10 years.

# CASE 9: ANAEMIA

## History

A 39-year-old woman is referred from the haematologist, with anaemia. She had been complaining of increasing tiredness and shortness of breath for 3 months, with frequent headaches.

Her periods occur every 24 days and the first day is generally moderate but the second to fourth days are very heavy. She uses tampons and sanitary towels together. She has no pain. Her last smear test was normal 2 years ago. She had no previous gynaecological problems and takes no medication.

## Examination

The woman is slim with pale conjunctivae. Abdominal, bimanual and speculum examination are unremarkable.

---

### INVESTIGATIONS

|  |  | Normal |
|---|---|---|
| Haemoglobin | 6.3 g/dL | 11.7–15.7 g/dL |
| Mean cell volume | 66 fL | 80–99 fL |
| White cell count | $9.1 \times 10^9$/L | $3.5–11 \times 10^9$/L |
| Platelets | $300 \times 10^9$/L | $150–440 \times 10^9$/L |
| Ferritin | 9 µg/L | 6–81 µg/L |
| Iron | 7 µmol/L | 10–28 µmol/L |
| Total iron-binding capacity (TIBC) | 80 µmol/L | 45–72 µmol/L |

Blood film: hypochromic microcytic red cells

*Transvaginal ultrasound scan report (day 4):* the uterus is normal size and retroverted. The endometrium is smooth and thin measuring 3.1 mm. Both ovaries are normal.

---

## Questions

- How do you interpret these findings?
- What is the likely underlying diagnosis?
- How would you manage this woman?

# ANSWER 9

The blood count shows anaemia with reduced mean cell corpuscular volume and low mean cell haemoglobin suggestive of a microcytic anaemia. Iron deficiency is the commonest cause for this picture and is confirmed by the low ferritin and iron, with raised iron-binding capacity. The anaemia accounts for the breathlessness, tiredness and headaches.

Menorrhagia is the commonest cause of anaemia in women, and in this case is supported by the history of excessive bleeding. The woman herself may not recognize that her periods are particularly heavy if she has always experienced heavy periods or if she thinks it is normal for periods to become heavier as she gets older.

As no other cause of heavy bleeding is apparent from the history and the ultrasound is normal, then the underlying diagnosis is one of exclusion referred to as dysfunctional uterine bleeding (DUB).

---

**!**    **Dysfunctional uterine bleeding**

Excessive heavy, prolonged or frequent bleeding that is not due to pregnancy or any recognizable pelvic or systemic disease

---

## Management

The anaemia should be treated with ferrous sulphate 200 mg twice daily until haemoglobin and ferritin are normal. It may take 3–6 months for iron stores to be fully replenished. Tranexamic acid (an antifibrinolytic) should be given during menstruation to reduce the amount of bleeding. It is contraindicated with a history of thromboembolic disease.

The levonorgestrel-releasing intrauterine device is used for its action on the endometrium to reduce menorrhagia, often causing amenorrhoea, though it is commonly associated with irregular bleeding for the first 3 months. The combined oral contraceptive pill is effective for menorrhagia in young women (below 35 years).

If these first-line management options are ineffective then endometrial ablation should be considered, which destroys the endometrium down to the basal layer. It is successful in 80–85 per cent of women and they should have completed their family and use effective contraception.

Hysterectomy is considered a 'last resort' for DUB, due to the associated morbidity.

---

 **KEY POINTS**

- A woman's perception of bleeding is not always proportionate to the actual volume lost, so haemoglobin should be checked in any woman suspected of menorrhagia.
- DUB is a diagnosis of exclusion.
- A hierarchy of first-, second- and third-line treatment should be used in management.

---

# CASE 10: ABSENT PERIODS

## History

A 24-year-old woman presents with the absence of periods for 9 months. She started her periods at the age of 13 years and had a regular 28-day cycle until 18 months ago. The periods then became irregular, occurring every 2–3 months until they stopped completely. She has also had headaches for the last few months and is not sure if this is related. She has a regular sexual partner and uses condoms for contraception. She has never been pregnant. There is no previous medical history of note.

She works as a primary school teacher and drinks approximately 4 units of alcohol per week. She does not smoke or use recreational drugs. She jogs and swims in her spare time.

## Examination

The woman is of average build. The blood pressure and general observations are normal. The abdomen is soft and non-tender and speculum and bimanual examination are unremarkable.

| INVESTIGATIONS | | |
|---|---|---|
| | | Normal |
| Follicle-stimulating hormone | 7 IU/L | Day 2–5 |
| | | 1–11 IU/L |
| Luteinizing hormone | 4 IU/L | Day 2–5 |
| | | 0.5–14.5 IU/L |
| Prolactin | 1800 mu/L | 90–520 mu/L |
| Testosterone | 1.8 nmol/L | 0.8–3.1 nmol/L |

Magnetic resonance imaging (MRI) scan of the head is shown in Fig. 10.1.

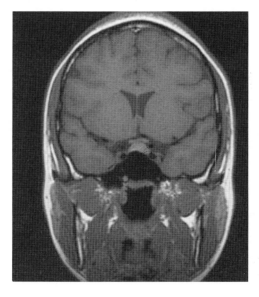

**Figure 10.1** MRI scan of the head.

## Questions
- What is the diagnosis?
- Are any further investigations indicated?
- How would you manage this patient?

# ANSWER 10

The investigations show a high-prolactin and a space-occupying lesion in the pituitary fossa in the region of the anterior pituitary as detailed in Figure 10.2. This is consistent with a pituitary adenoma (prolactinoma).

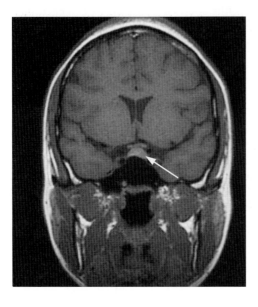

**Figure 10.2** Arrow shows a small asymmetrical enlargement of pituitary gland, representative of a small pituitary adenoma (prolactinoma).

Prolactin should always be measured in a woman with amenorrhoea. Care should be taken in interpreting the results, as levels up to 1000 mu/L can be found as a result of stress (even due to venepuncture), breast examination or in association with polycystic ovarian syndrome. Above 1000 mu/L the usual cause is a pituitary adenoma (micro- or macroscopic).

---

**!  Differential diagnosis of secondary amenorrhoea**

- *Hypothalamic*:
  - chronic illness
  - anorexia
  - excessive exercise
  - stress
- *Pituitary*:
  - hyperprolactinaemia (e.g. drugs, tumour)
  - hypothyroidism
  - breast-feeding
- *Ovarian*:
  - polycystic ovarian syndrome
  - premature ovarian failure
  - iatrogenic (chemotherapy, radiotherapy, oophorectomy)
  - long-acting progesterone contraception
- *Uterine*:
  - pregnancy
  - Asherman's syndrome
  - cervical stenosis

---

## Further investigation

Visual fields should be checked, as visual field defects may be present with a large tumour. The other important investigation in any woman with amenorrhoea is a pregnancy test, although with this history this would be very unlikely. (Prolactin is also raised in pregnancy.)

## Management

Most prolactinomas respond to medical treatment with bromocriptine or cabergoline. Maintaining the prolactin level below 1000 mu/L causes menstruation (and ovulation) to return in most women. This can be continued indefinitely or until pregnancy is achieved if the presenting complaint is of infertility.

 **KEY POINTS**

- Hyperprolactinaemia is a common cause of secondary amenorrhoea.
- Prolactin levels up to 1000 u/L may be due to non-pathological causes such as stress.
- Prolactinomas can usually be treated with medical suppression, and surgery is only indicated rarely.

# CASE 11: POSTMENOPAUSAL BLEEDING

## History

A 59-year-old woman awoke with blood on her nightdress, which was bright red but not heavy. There were no clots of blood and there was no associated pain. The bleeding has recurred twice since in similar amounts.

Her last period was at the age of 49 years and she has had no other intervening bleeding episodes. She suffered hot flushes and night sweats around the time of her menopause, which have now stopped. She is sexually active but has noticed vaginal dryness on intercourse recently.

She has always had normal cervical smears, the last one being 7 months ago. She had two children by spontaneous vaginal delivery and had a laparoscopic sterilization aged 34 years. She has never used hormone-replacement therapy (HRT). She takes atenolol for hypertension and omeprazole for epigastric pain.

## Examination

She is slightly overweight. Abdominal examination is normal. The vulva and vagina appear thin and atrophic and the cervix is normal. The uterus is small and anteverted and with no palpable adnexal masses.

An outpatient endometrial biopsy is taken at the time of examination and sent for histological examination.

|  INVESTIGATIONS |
| :--- |
| Transvaginal ultrasound scan is shown in Fig. 11.1. |
| *Endometrial biopsy report*: the specimen shows atrophic endometrium with no evidence of inflammation, hyperplasia or malignancy. |

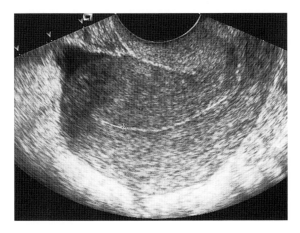

Figure 11.1 Transvaginal ultrasound scan.

## Questions

- What is the likely diagnosis?
- How would you manage this patient?

# ANSWER 11

Postmenopausal bleeding is considered to be caused by endometrial cancer until proven otherwise. However, only 10 per cent of women with postmenopausal bleeding are diagnosed with endometrial cancer.

---

**!**  **Causes of postmenopausal bleeding**

- Endometrial cancer
- Endometrial/endocervical polyp
- Endometrial hyperplasia
- Atrophic vaginitis
- Iatrogenic (anticoagulants, intrauterine device, hormone-replacement therapy)
- Infective (vaginal candidiasis)

---

In this case the endometrium is <5 mm on ultrasound, which effectively excludes an endometrial malignancy or polyp. The normal endometrial biopsy report confirms the absence of endometrial pathology. The smear history is normal, and the cervix appears normal, excluding cervical cancer. She is not taking any medication that may predispose to abnormal bleeding.

The diagnosis of atrophic vaginitis can therefore be made by exclusion of serious causes, and is backed up by the history of vaginal dryness at sexual intercourse and the atrophic vulva and vagina noted on examination.

## Management

Treatment is hormonal with a course of topical oestrogen given daily for 3 weeks and then twice weekly for maintenance, for an initial period of 2-3 months. An alternative solution is to give a combined form of systemic HRT to protect the endometrium.

Some women are reluctant to use HRT because of the associated risks, and therefore advice should be given about vaginal lubricants which decrease discomfort but have no reparative value. If bleeding recurs after treatment or the diagnosis is in doubt, then further investigation with hysteroscopy and dilatation and curettage is needed.

---

  KEY POINTS

- Women with postmenopausal bleeding (PMB) should be considered to have endometrial cancer until proven otherwise.
- Endometrial thickness, endometrial biopsy and hysteroscopy are used to investigate PMB.
- Atrophic vaginitis can be treated with courses of topical oestrogens

---

# CASE 12: PAINFUL PERIODS

## History

A 43-year-old woman is referred from her general practitioner (GP) with painful periods. She says that her periods have always been quite heavy and painful but that in the last 2–3 years they have become almost unbearable. She bleeds every 24 days and the period lasts for 7–9 days with very heavy flow from day 2 to day 6. The pain starts approximately 36 h before the onset of the bleeding and lasts until about day 5. The pain is constant, dull and severe, such that she cannot do any housework or any social activities during this time. Her GP has prescribed paracetamol and mefenamic acid in combination, which she says 'takes the edge off' but does not fully relieve the symptoms.

She has had four normal deliveries and her husband had a vasectomy several years ago.

There is no history of intermenstrual or postcoital discharge and she has no abnormal discharge. Her smear history is normal, the most recent being 18 months ago. She takes citalopram for depression but currently reports her mood as fine. She does not drink alcohol or smoke.

## Examination

The abdomen is soft and there is vague tenderness in the suprapubic area. The cervix appears normal. On bimanual palpation the uterus is approximately 10 weeks size, soft and bulky. She is tender on palpation but there is no cervical excitation, adnexal tenderness or adnexal masses.

---

### 🔍 INVESTIGATIONS

Transvaginal ultrasound scan is shown in Fig. 12.1

*Transvaginal ultrasound report*: there is asymmetrical uterine enlargement, with a thickened posterior uterine wall. There are ill-defined cystic spaces within the posterior myometrial wall. There is an indistinct myometrial–endometrial border. Both ovaries appear normal in size and morphology.

---

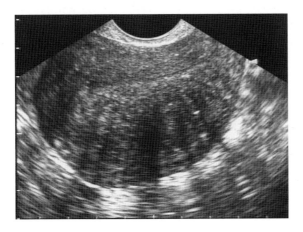

Figure 12.1 Transvaginal ultrasound scan of the uterus.

## Questions
- What is the likely diagnosis?
- How would you further investigate and manage this woman?

# ANSWER 12

The symptoms of dysmenorrhoea and menorrhagia and the ultrasound report suggest a diagnosis of adenomyosis. This is a benign condition whereby functioning endometrial glands and stroma are found within the myometrium. With each period bleeding occurs from the endometrial tissue into the smooth muscle, with associated pain. It tends to occur in women over 35 years and risk factors include increased parity, termination and previous Caesarean section. The condition may commonly be found in association with endometriosis. Classically the diagnosis may only be made histologically after hysterectomy for dysmenorrhoea. More recently however the diagnosis can be suspected by ultrasound or magnetic resonance imaging (MRI) scan.

---

**!  Causes of dysmenorrhoea**

- Idiopathic
- Premenstrual syndrome
- Pelvic inflammatory disease
- Endometriosis
- Adenomyosis
- Submucosal pedunculated fibroids
- Iatrogenic (e.g. intrauterine contraceptive device (IUCD) or cervical stenosis after large-loop excision of the transformation zone (LLETZ))

---

## Further investigation

If the diagnosis is in doubt then an MRI scan may be requested. Hysterectomy to obtain histological diagnosis would be inappropriate.

## Management

The initial management involves analgesia such as mefenamic acid and codydramol. Tranexamic acid reduces the amount of bleeding and this may secondarily reduce the amount of pain. Suppression of menstruation with gonadotrophin-releasing hormone analogues is a short-term measure. The levonorgestrel-releasing intrauterine device is another option to locally suppress the endometrial tissue, and may resolve the pain.

As a last resort hysterectomy should be performed.

---

  **KEY POINTS**

- The prevalence of adenomyosis is unknown, as diagnosis is only confirmed by hysterectomy.
- It is a cause of menorrhagia and dysmenorrhoea in older women.
- Hysterectomy may be avoided by use of analgesia or hormonal suppression.

---

# CASE 13: POSTCOITAL BLEEDING

## History

An 18-year-old woman is referred with postcoital bleeding. It has occurred on approximately seven occasions over the preceding 6 weeks. Generally it has been a small amount of bright red blood noticed a few hours after intercourse and lasting up to 2 days. There is no associated pain.

Her last menstrual period started 3 weeks ago and she bleeds for 4 days every 28 days. Her periods were previously quite heavy but are now lighter since she started the combined oral contraceptive pill (COCP) 6 months ago. There is no history of an abnormal discharge or offensive odour and she has no dyspareunia.

She has had three sexual partners and has been with her current partner for 10 months. She has never been diagnosed with any sexually transmitted infection and has never had a smear test. She had an appendectomy at the age of 7 years and was diagnosed with epilepsy in childhood but has been off all medication for 8 years.

## Examination

The abdomen is soft and non-tender. Speculum examination reveals a florid reddened area symmetrically surrounding the external cervical os with contact bleeding. The uterus is normal sized, anteverted and non-tender. There is no cervical excitation and the adnexae are unremarkable.

## Questions
- What is the differential diagnosis?
- What further investigations would you perform for this woman?
- If your investigations are negative what is the likely diagnosis and how would you manage the woman?

# ANSWER 13

Postcoital bleeding in a young woman is common and normally benign. In this specific case the examination findings are consistent only with cervical ectropion, malignancy or infection.

---

**!** **Differential diagnoses of postcoital bleeding in a young woman**

- Cervical ectropion
- Chlamydia or other sexually transmitted infection (STI)
- Cervical malignancy
- Complication of the COCP
- Endocervical polyp

---

## Investigations

An STI screen should be performed:

- endocervical swab for chlamydia
- endocervical swab for gonorrhoea
- high vaginal swab for trichomonas (and candida, not a STI, but possibly a cause of irregular bleeding from vaginitis).

A cervical smear should also be taken to exclude cervical intraepithelial neoplasia or malignancy prior to treatment.

## Management

Assuming the swabs and smear are negative then the diagnosis is of cervical ectropion. This is particularly common around the time of puberty, in women using the COCP, and in pregnancy. It is not of clinical significance and is generally an incidental finding but warrants treatment if it causes embarrassing and troublesome bleeding (or discharge in some cases).

There are three options for treatment:

1. stop the COCP and use alternative contraception
2. cold coagulation of the cervix
3. diathermy ablation of the ectocervix.

---

 **KEY POINTS**

- Cervical ectropion is very common and usually incidental and asymptomatic.
- It occurs particularly in pregnancy and with use of the COCP.
- Postcoital bleeding should always be investigated to exclude significant pathology.

---

# CASE 14: RECURRENT MISCARRIAGE

## History

A 34-year-old woman is referred from the emergency room with vaginal bleeding at 6 weeks and 5 days' gestation. Bleeding started 2 days ago and was initially spotting but has now increased so that she needs to change a sanitary towel regularly. There is a mild dull lower abdominal pain.

She normally has regular 28-day cycle. In the past she has used the combined oral contraceptive pill but stopped 3 years ago when she and her partner decided to start a family.

She is gravida 3 para 0. Her first pregnancy ended in a complete miscarriage 2 years ago. Five months ago she had a missed miscarriage at 9 weeks and required ERPC (evacuation of retained products of conception).

There is no gynaecological history of note. Medically she is fit and healthy, except for mild asthma for which she takes inhalers.

The woman's mother died from a pulmonary embolism after her last child. Her brother also had a deep venous thrombosis at the age of 29 years. Her sister has two children, both born preterm because of severe pre-eclampsia.

## Examination

The abdomen is non-distended but tender suprapubically. The cervical os is open and products of conception are removed from the os and sent for histological examination.

The bleeding subsequently settles.

---

### 🔍 INVESTIGATIONS

| | | Normal range for pregnancy |
|---|---|---|
| Haemoglobin | 11.1 g/dL | 11–14 g/dL |
| White cell count | $3.9 \times 10^9$/L | $6–16 \times 10^9$/L |
| Platelets | $201 \times 10^9$/L | $150–400 \times 10^9$/L |

Anticardiolipin antibody: positive

Lupus anticoagulant: positive

*Histology report*: chorionic villi are seen, confirming products of conception.

---

## Questions

- What is the likely underlying diagnosis for the recurrent miscarriages?
- What further investigation should be performed?
- How should this patient be managed?

# ANSWER 14

Raised anticardiolipin antibodies and lupus anticoagulant are suggestive of antiphospholipid syndrome.

---

| ! | Diagnosis of antiphospholipid syndrome |
|---|---|

- The presence of one of the clinical features:
  - three or more consecutive miscarriages
  - mid-trimester fetal loss
  - severe early-onset pre-eclampsia, intrauterine growth restriction or abruption
  - arterial or venous thrombosis
- *And* haematological features:
  - anticardiolipin antibody or lupus anticoagulant detected on two occasions at least 6 weeks apart

---

Thus in this case the diagnosis must be confirmed by a second positive anticardiolipin test after at least 6 weeks. She should also be tested for antinuclear and anti-double-stranded DNA antibodies as antiphospholipid syndrome is often secondary to systemic lupus erythematosus (SLE).

## Management

Oral low-dose aspirin and low-molecular-weight subcutaneous heparin from the time of a positive pregnancy test should be given in subsequent pregnancies to improve the likelihood of a successful live birth.

Psychological support should be given with regular reassurance ultrasound scans in the first trimester. There is evidence that shows repeated ultrasound scans for reassurance alone improve the outcome after recurrent miscarriage.

---

| ! | Causes of recurrent miscarriage |
|---|---|

- Parental chromosome abnormality (3–5 per cent, e.g. balanced chromosomal abnormality)
- Antiphospholipid syndrome
- Other thrombophilia (e.g. activated protein C resistance)
- Uterine abnormality (intracavity fibroids, uterine septum)
- Uncontrolled diabetes or hypothyroidism
- Bacterial vaginosis (usually associated with second-trimester loss)
- Cervical weakness ('incompetence', second-trimester loss only)

---

| 🔑 | KEY POINTS |
|---|---|

- Only a minority of women with recurrent miscarriage will have a cause identified.
- Aspirin and heparin are effective in women with antiphospholipid syndrome.
- Reassurance ultrasound scans and support improve outcome for women with recurrent loss.

---

## CASE 15: PELVIC PAIN

### History

A 29-year-old woman presents with lower abdominal pain for 4 years occurring with her periods. She takes paracetamol and ibuprofen and goes to bed with a hot water bottle for up to 2 days every month. For the last 18 months pain has also occurred in between periods.

The pain is dull and constant across the lower abdomen. Her periods are regular and there is no menorrhagia, intermenstrual or postcoital bleeding. There is no other significant medical history.

She has been married for 2 years and has deep dyspareunia which makes her interrupt intercourse. She does not use any contraception, as they are keen to start a family. She has never been pregnant in the past.

### Examination

There is generalized lower-abdominal tenderness, particularly in the suprapubic area but no masses are palpable. Speculum examination is unremarkable. On bimanual palpation the uterus is axial and fixed with cervical excitation. The pouch of Douglas is very tender and contains a mass. The adnexae are both tender but no adnexal masses are palpable.

---

 **INVESTIGATIONS**

Transvaginal ultrasound scan is shown in Fig. 15.1.

The findings at laparoscopy are shown in Fig. 15.2.

---

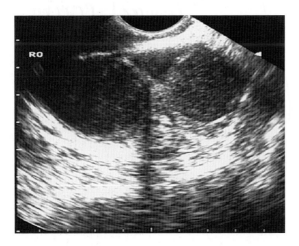

**Figure 15.1** Transvaginal ultrasound scan.

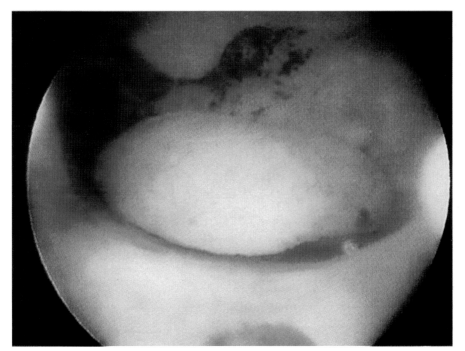

Plate 1   Fig. 1.2 Hysteroscopic appearance of endometrial polyp prior to resection. Case 1 Intermenstrual bleeding, p 2.

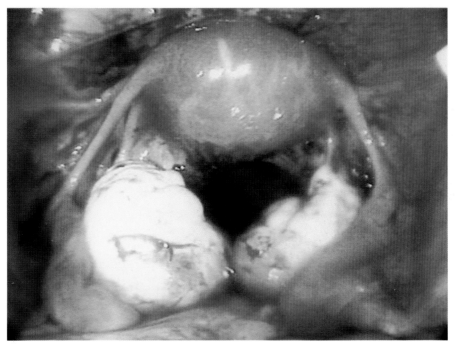

Plate 2   Fig. 15.2 Findings at laparoscopy. Case 15 Pelvic pain, p 37.

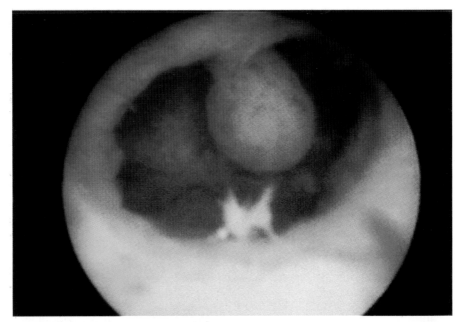

Plate 3  Fig. 17.1 Hysteroscopy. Case 17 Heavy periods, p 43.

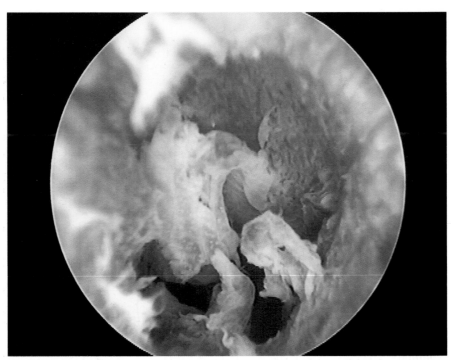

Plate 4  Fig. 22.1 Hysteroscopy findings. Case 22 Postmenopausal bleeding, p 55.

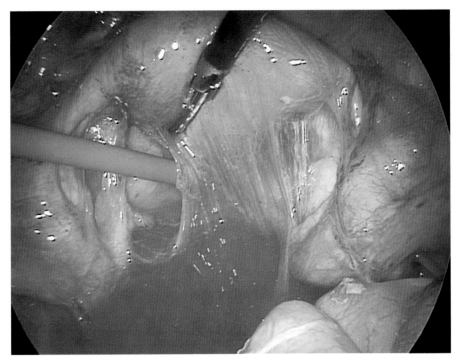

Plate 5 Fig. 23.1 Laparoscopy findings. Case 23 Pelvic pain, p 58.

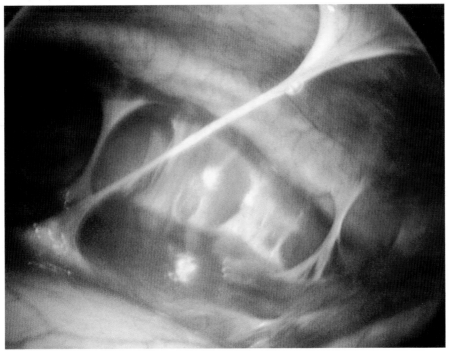

Plate 6 Fig. 23.2 Laparoscopy findings. Case 23, Pelvic pain, p 59.

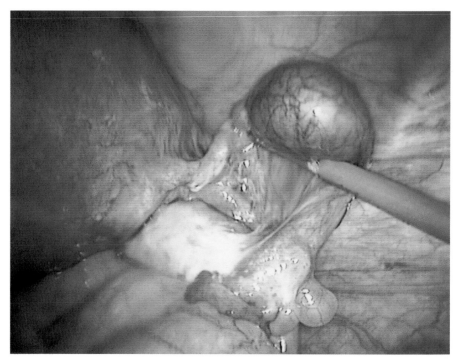

Plate 7 Fig. 41.2 Laparoscopy findings. Case 41 Bleeding and pain in early pregnancy, p 99.

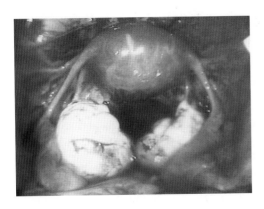

**Figure 15.2** Findings at laparoscopy. See Plate 2 for colour image.

## Questions

- What is the diagnosis?
- How would you further manage this woman?

# ANSWER 15

The history of dysmenorrhoea and dyspareunia are classic for endometriosis, and the ultrasound examination and laparoscopy images show bilateral endometriomas ('chocolate cysts'), a complication of this disease.

Endometriosis is a common condition where active endometrial glands and stroma are located outside the endometrial cavity. Endometriomas develop as ectopic endometrial tissue on the ovary produces blood, which builds up into an encapsulated cyst with each consecutive menstrual cycle.

Endometriosis is benign but carries a high physical and psychological morbidity due to the clinical features:

- pelvic pain
- dysmenorrhoea
- dyspareunia
- infertility.

Examination findings include tenderness or a pelvic mass, and may include palpable nodules in the rectovaginal septum and a fixed retroverted uterus secondary to adhesions (the frozen pelvis).

Diagnosis is made at laparoscopy, although ultrasound features such as these ovarian cysts containing 'ground-glass' echoes can be suggestive.

## Management

The mainstay of management for endometriosis is surgical, with ablation or excision of endometriotic deposits by laparoscopy. In this case there are bilateral endometriotic cysts that need to be removed laparoscopically by incision and drainage with excision of the cyst capsules. Surgical treatment should relieve the dyspareunia and dysmenorrhoea and may improve fertility in more severe disease.

Medical suppression of endometriosis is possible with the contraceptive pill or gonadotrophin-releasing hormone analogues, which inhibit ovulation and hence stimulation of endometrial deposits by oestrogen. However these are ineffective for endometriomas. The levonorgestrel-releasing intrauterine device has also been used to suppress endometriosis and reduce symptoms.

---

 **KEY POINTS**

- Endometriosis classically presents with dysmenorrhoea, dyspareunia and infertility.
- Endometriosis is often diagnosed years after symptoms start.
- Surgical excision is the mainstay of treatment.

# CASE 16: INFERTILITY

## History

A 31-year-old woman and her 34-year-old partner are referred by the general practitioner because of primary infertility. They have been trying to conceive for over 2 years. The woman has regular menstrual periods bleeding for 4 days every 28–30 days. Her periods are not heavy and have never been painful. There is no intermenstrual bleeding or discharge and no postcoital bleeding. She has never been diagnosed with any sexually transmitted infections.

The last smear was normal 1 year ago. She is a non-smoker and drinks alcohol very occasionally.

The partner's only previous medical history was an appendectomy and a course of anti-helicobacter therapy after he developed epigastric pain and was diagnosed with the infection. He previously smoked 20 cigarettes per day and drank up to 28 units of alcohol per week but has now stopped smoking and significantly reduced his alcohol intake. He works as buyer for a retail company.

The couple have intercourse 1–4 times per week and there is no reported sexual dysfunction or pain on intercourse. They both deny recreational drug use.

## Examination

On examination the woman has a body mass index of $23 \, \text{kg/m}^2$. There is no hirsutism or acne. There are no signs of thyroid disease. The abdomen is soft and non-tender. Speculum and bimanual palpation are unremarkable. Genital examination of the partner is also normal.

---

### 🔍 INVESTIGATIONS

|  |  | Normal |
|---|---|---|
| Follicle-stimulating hormone (day 3) | 4.2 IU/L | Day 2–5 |
|  |  | 1–11 IU/L |
| Luteinizing hormone (day 3) | 2.7 IU/L | Day 2–5 |
|  |  | 0.5–14.5 IU/L |
| Day 21 progesterone | 45 nmol/L |  |
| Prolactin | 374 mu/L | 90–520 mu/L |
| Testosterone | 2.0 nmol/L | 0.8–3.1 nmol/L |
| *Semen analysis*: |  |  |
| Volume | 4 mL | 2–5 mL |
| Count | 63 million/mL | >20 million/mL |
| Normal forms | 22 per cent | >15 per cent normal shape |
| Motility | 53 per cent progressively mobile | >50 per cent progressively mobile |

Rubella antibody: immune

Chlamydia: negative

A hysterosalpingogram is shown in Fig. 16.1.

---

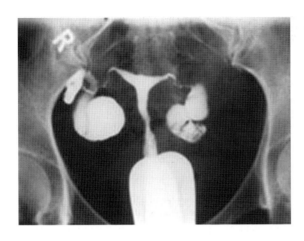

**Figure 16.1** Hysterosalpingogram.

**Questions**
- How do you interpret the investigation results?
- Are any further investigations necessary?
- How would you manage this couple?

# ANSWER 16

Day 21 progesterone above 30 nmol/L confirms ovulation, and this is supported by normal follicle-stimulating hormone (FSH), luteinizing hormone (LH) and prolactin. Normal testosterone suggests that polycystic ovaries is an unlikely diagnosis.

The semen analysis is normal, and therefore any male factor aetiology is unlikely. Rubella immunity should always be confirmed.

The hysterosalpingogram shows fill of contrast medium into both uterine tubes but no spill, suggesting tubal obstruction as the cause of the fertility problem.

## Further investigations

Tubal blockage on hysterosalpinogram can sometimes be due to tubal spasm, and therefore a laparoscopy and dye is needed to confirm the pathology and also to determine a cause such as adhesions from previous infection or possibly endometriosis (although the history does not support this diagnosis).

## Management

If the tubes are found at dye test to be patent, then this would suggest that it is feasible to attempt pregnancy with in utero insemination. However if blocked tubes are confirmed then in vitro fertilization (IVF) is indicated. Abnormal tubes are usually removed prior to IVF, as success rates for pregnancy are better and ectopic pregnancy rate reduced after bilateral salpingectomy.

General advice should be given to take folic acid 400 µg daily to reduce the risk of neural tube defects, and to the partner to minimize his alcohol intake.

In this case the laparoscopy showed bilateral hydrosalpinges and adhesions as well as perihepatic 'violin-string' adhesions. These findings are consistent with previous infection with chlamydia (or more rarely gonorrhoea). It is not unusual to find such severe pelvic adhesions even when there has never been a clear clinical history of pelvic infection or sexually transmitted infection. Although the infection may be long ago, it is sensible to treat both the woman and her partner with a course of antibiotics for pelvic inflammatory disease.

---

 **KEY POINTS**

- Infertility may be due to anovulation, tubal or endometrial/uterine pathology as well as male factors.
- Up to 30 per cent of infertile couples have more than one factor causing infertility.
- Tubal obstruction on hysterosalpingogram is not always confirmed at laparoscopy.

# CASE 17: HEAVY PERIODS

## History

A 39-year-old woman complains of increasingly long and heavy periods over the last 5 years. Previously she bled for 4 days but now bleeding lasts up to 10 days. The periods still occur every 28 days. She experiences intermenstrual bleeding between most periods but no postcoital bleeding.

The periods were never painful previously but in recent months have become extremely painful with intermittent cramps. She has had four normal deliveries and had a laparoscopic sterilization after her last child. Her smear tests have always been normal, the most recent being 4 months ago. She has never had any previous irregular bleeding or any other gynaecological problems.

## Examination

The abdomen is soft and non-tender with no palpable masses. Speculum examination shows a normal cervix. On bimanual palpation the uterus is bulky (approximately 8 week size), mobile and anteverted. There are no adnexal masses.

---

### 🔍 INVESTIGATIONS

|  |  | Normal range |
| --- | --- | --- |
| Haemoglobin | 9.2 g/dL | 11.7–15.7 g/dL |
| Mean cell volume | 75 fL | 80–99 fL |
| White cell count | $4.5 \times 10^9$/L | $3.5–11 \times 10^9$/L |
| Platelets | $198 \times 10^9$/L | $150–440 \times 10^9$/L |

Findings at hysteroscopy are shown in Fig. 17.1.

---

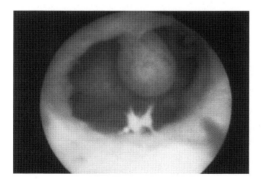

Figure 17.1 Hysteroscopy. See Plate 3 for colour image.

## Questions
- What is the diagnosis?
- How would you manage this patient and counsel her about the management and its potential risks?

# ANSWER 17

The ultrasound scan shows a submucosal fibroid and this is confirmed by the hysteroscopy image. At hysteroscopy, a fibroid is a solid smooth immobile structure, whereas a polyp appears pink and fleshy and mobile. Submucosal fibroids are a common cause of menorrhagia and can cause, as in this case, intermenstrual bleeding. The cramp-like pain occurs as the uterus tries to expel the fibroid. In some cases this eventually occurs with the fibroid becoming pedunculated and extending through to the vagina on a pedicle.

## Management

The management is by hysteroscopic (transcervical) resection of the fibroid (TCRF). This can be performed as a day case under general anaesthetic (or even local anaesthetic if the fibroid is small). The important points in counselling the patient are as follows.

- *Description of the procedure*: the procedure involves stretching (dilatation) of the cervix and insertion of an endoscope into the uterus (hysteroscopy) to view the fibroid. The fibroid is 'shaved' away with a hot wire loop (diathermy). Fluid is circulated through the uterine cavity to enhance the view and allow cooling.
- *What are the risks?*
  - bleeding: it is rare to bleed heavily but in the extreme situation blood transfusion could be required, or even a hysterectomy to control the loss
  - infection
  - fluid overload: during the procedure, irrigation fluid is absorbed into the circulation. Excessive absorption can cause breathing difficulties (pulmonary oedema) and the need for hospital admission
  - uterine perforation: rarely the hysteroscope perforates the wall of the uterus and if this occurs or is suspected then laparoscopy is needed immediately to confirm it, secure any bleeding and check for damage to surrounding bowel or bladder.
- *What to expect afterwards*: most women experience bleeding, discharge and passing of 'debris' for up to 2 weeks after the procedure.

---

 KEY POINTS

- Ultrasound is critical in the diagnosis of menorrhagia.
- Submucosal fibroids are more likely to cause menorrhagia than those that are intramural or subserous.
- Transcervical resection of fibroids is a relatively simple procedure but is associated with important risks.

---

# CASE 18: URINARY INCONTINENCE

## History

A 61-year-old woman complains of involuntary loss of urine. She has noticed it gradually over the last 10 years and has finally decided to see her general practitioner about it after hearing a programme on the radio about treatment for incontinence. The leaking is generally small amounts and she wears a pad all the time. It tends to occur when she cannot get to the toilet in time. She never leaks on coughing or sneezing. She suffers urgency, particularly when she comes home after being out and is about to come into the house. She also has frequency, passing urine every hour during the day and getting up two or three times each night.

Due to the incontinence she tries not to drink much and usually has two cups of tea first thing in the morning, coffee mid-morning and a further cup of tea mid-afternoon. Other than that she drinks one glass of squash per day and has one glass of wine at night.

She is a non-smoker. She has had two uncomplicated vaginal deliveries. Her periods stopped at the age of 54 years. There is no other gynaecological or medical history of note.

## Examination

Abdominal examination is normal. On vaginal examination there is minimal uterovaginal descent and no anterior or posterior vaginal wall prolapse.

---

 **INVESTIGATIONS**

Midstream urinalysis: protein negative, blood negative, leucocytes negative, nitrites negative

*Urodynamics*: the first urge to void was reported at 150 mL bladder filling. Involuntary detrusor contractions were noted while the patient was attempting to inhibit micturition. There was no loss of urine with coughing.

---

## Questions
- What is the diagnosis?
- How would you advise and manage this patient?

# ANSWER 18

The diagnosis is of overactive bladder syndrome (OAB). This was formerly referred to as detrusor instability. In this condition the bladder contracts involuntarily without the normal trigger to void caused by bladder filling. This results in involuntary loss of urine that is embarrassing and often impacts enormously on women's lives, as they are constantly aware of needing to void and where the nearest toilet might be.

Urodynamic investigation with filling and voiding cystometry is helpful (as in this case) in confirming the diagnosis by showing spontaneous detrusor contractions during bladder filling.

It is important to exclude other causes of such symptoms (such as urinary tract infection or a bladder tumour) with urine microscopy.

## Management
- *Conservative*:
  - the woman should be advised that both caffeine and alcohol are bladder stimulants and are likely to worsen symptoms so should be minimized. She should take a normal fluid intake per day but avoid drinks after about 7 pm to limit nocturia
  - bladder retraining for 6 weeks, involving a 'drill' restricting voiding to increasing intervals should be taught.
- *Medical treatment*: if lifestyle advice and bladder retraining fail then anticholinergic medication such as oxybutynin or tolterodine should be commenced. The associated side-effects include dry mouth, dry eyes and constipation.

---

 | **KEY POINTS**

- Overactive bladder syndrome is associated with urgency, frequency and urge incontinence.
- Conservative measures are bladder retraining and caffeine avoidance.
- Medical treatment is with anticholinergics.

---

# CASE 19: ABSENT PERIODS

## History

An 18-year-old woman presents with an absence of periods for 6 months. This has occurred twice before in the past but on both occasions menstruation returned so she was not too concerned. Her periods started at the age of 12 years and were initially regular. She has no medical history of note and denies any medication. She is currently in her first year at university. She runs most days and reports a 'healthy' diet avoiding carbohydrate foods and meat. She is the oldest of three siblings and her parents separated when she was 12 years. She has minimal contact with her father and lives mainly with her mother who she says she gets on well with. She has had a boyfriend in the past but has veered away from any sexual relationships.

## Examination

The woman is tall and thin with a body mass index (BMI) of 15.5 kg/m$^2$. There is evidence of fine downy hair growth on her arms. Heart rate is 86/min and blood pressure 100/65 mmHg. Abdominal examination reveals no scars or masses, and genital examination is not performed.

| INVESTIGATIONS | | |
|---|---|---|
| | | *Normal* |
| Follicle-stimulating hormone | 1.0 IU/L | Day 2–5 |
| | | 1–11 IU/L |
| Luteinizing hormone | 0.8 IU/L | Day 2–5 |
| | | 0.5–14.5 IU/L |
| Oestradiol | 52 pmol/L | 70–600 pmol/L |
| Prolactin | 630 mu/L | 90–520 mu/L |
| Testosterone | 1.6 nmol/L | 0.8–3.1 nmol/L |

## Questions
- What is the diagnosis?
- How would you further investigate and manage this woman?

# ANSWER 19

The woman has evidence of hypogonadotrophic hypogonadism – she has low oestradiol levels associated with low gonadotrophin stimulation from the anterior pituitary. This may be due to various pituitary or hypothalamic causes, but in this case clearly relates to anorexia nervosa and possibly excessive exercise. The raised prolactin is consistent with stress and does not need to be investigated further. At a BMI below $18 \, kg/m^2$, menstruation tends to cease, returning once the BMI increases again.

The previous episodes of amenorrhoea probably occurred when her dietary intake was very low and it may be that starting at university may have increased her stress levels with the consequence of worsening her anorexia.

## Further investigation
- Full blood count, liver and renal function should all be monitored as these are affected in severe disease.
- A bone scan should be arranged to check for bone density – hypo-oestrogenism as a result of anorexia is likely to induce early-onset osteoporosis and fractures.
- Pyschological assessment is also important to guide appropriate treatment.

## Management
Encouraging the woman to eat a more normal diet and to avoid exercising is the ideal management, but anorexia is a chronic disease that is often refractory to treatment. Explanation that her periods will return if she increases her BMI may possibly encourage her to put on weight.

The combined oral contraceptive pill should be prescribed in the meantime, which will prevent osteoporosis and bring on periods, albeit pharmacologically induced.

Referral to a specialist eating disorders unit is vital in addressing the long-term problem for this woman. Commonly, eating disorders arise out of childhood difficulties and family or group therapy should be considered.

If the investigations suggest renal or hepatic impairment then inpatient management is likely to be necessary.

---

 **KEY POINTS**

- Menstruation usually ceases when BMI is less than $18 \, kg/m^2$.
- Amenorrhoeic anorexic women need oestrogen replacement to protect them from osteoporosis.
- Anorexia is often refractory to treatment.

---

## CASE 20: ABDOMINAL AND BACK PAIN

### History

An 83-year-old woman complains of a dragging sensation in the lower abdomen and lower back pain when standing or walking. It has been present for some years but she can now only stand for a short time before feeling uncomfortable. It is not noticeable at night. She has had four vaginal deliveries. She had her menopause at 52 years and took hormone-replacement therapy for several years for vasomotor symptoms. She has not had any postmenopausal bleeding and has not had a smear for several years.

She is generally constipated and sometimes finds she can only defecate by placing her fingers into the vagina and compressing a 'bulge' she can feel. She has mild frequency and gets up twice most nights to pass urine. There is no dysuria or haematuria. Occasionally she does not get to the toilet in time and leaks a small amount of urine, but this does not worry her unduly.

Medically she is very well and does not take any medications regularly. She lives alone and does her own shopping and housework.

### Examination

On examination she appears well. Blood pressure and heart rate are normal. She is of average build. The abdomen is soft and non-tender. There is a loss of vulval anatomy consistent with atrophic changes. On examination in the supine position there is a mild prolapse. On standing, the cervix is felt at the level of the introitus. There is a large posterior wall prolapse and a minimal anterior wall prolapse.

### Questions
- What is the diagnosis for her discomfort and pain?
- How would you manage this patient?

# ANSWER 20

The diagnosis is of second-degree uterovaginal prolapse with rectocoele. Prolapse is traditionally categorized according to the level of descent of the cervix in relation to the introitus:

- *first degree*: descent within the vagina
- *second degree*: descent to the introitus
- *third degree*: descent of the cervix outside the vagina
- *procidentia*: complete eversion of the vagina outside the introitus.

More complex grading systems are used by some specialists that involve specific measurements using the hymen as a reference point.

Common presenting symptoms are of 'something coming down', a 'lump' or a dragging sensation. Symptoms are always worse on standing or walking because of the effect of gravity. Prolapse is more common in women who are parous, have had long or traumatic deliveries, have a chronic cough or constipation. However it may occur in any woman, even if she is nulliparous, as it relates to collagen strength.

## Management

Initial management involves treating the constipation with dietary manipulation and laxatives. This may relieve some of the symptoms and is also important to prevent recurrence if surgery is to be performed.

Pelvic floor exercises are helpful for mild prolapse and to preserve the integrity of repair postoperatively, though in this case they are unlikely to make any significant difference to the presenting symptoms. If surgery is not wanted then she can try a ring pessary to hold up the prolapse, which can work extremely well and only needs replacing every 6 months.

Although she is 83 this woman has no medical problems and should be offered definitive prolapse surgery which for her involves vaginal hysterectomy and posterior vaginal wall repair (colporrhaphy). As there is no abdominal incision involved, recovery is quick and she would expect to be in hospital for around 3 days.

---

 **KEY POINTS**

- Prolapse incidence increases with age, parity, constipation and chronic cough.
- Conservative management with a ring pessary, or surgical prolapse repair may be appropriate.
- Relief of exacerbating factors is important to prevent symptoms worsening or to maintain the integrity of the repair.

## CASE 21: POSTOPERATIVE CONFUSION

### History

You are on call and are asked to see a woman in the day surgery unit who is confused postoperatively. She is 42 years old and underwent transcervical resection of multiple submucosal fibroids in the early afternoon after presenting with menorrhagia. Four fibroids were resected and the estimated blood loss was 150 mL.

### Examination

The woman knows her name but is disorientated, scoring only 5/10 on a mini mental state examination. She seems slightly drowsy.

The heart rate is 100/min and the blood pressure is 105/70 mmHg. Oxygen saturation is 94 per cent on air. She is apyrexial. Chest examination reveals dullness at both bases with fine inspiratory crackles. The abdomen is not distended but there is generalized lower abdominal tenderness. No masses are palpable and there are no signs of peritonism. You can see that there is small amount of blood from the vagina, but the loss is not excessive. You are told that she passed urine an hour ago without difficulty.

The operation note is reviewed and you find that the procedure was essentially uncomplicated but was halted before all the fibroids could be fully resected because of the fluid imbalance. The fluid deficit is recorded as 1010 mL. However you review the actual fluid chart and it is as follows:

*Fluid input (glycine, via operating hysteroscope input channel):*

1000 mL

1000 mL

1000 mL

950 mL

*Fluid output (via operating hysteroscope output channel):*

1940 mL

---

### INVESTIGATIONS

|  |  | Normal |
|---|---|---|
| Haemoglobin | 10.4 g/dL | 11.7–15.7 g/dL |
| White cell count | 7.1 × 10⁹/L | 3.5–11 × 10⁹/L |
| Platelets | 302 × 10⁹/L | 150–440 × 10⁹/L |
| Sodium | 129 mmol/L | 135–145 mmol/L |
| Potassium | 3.1 mmol/L | 3.5–5 mmol/L |
| Urea | 1.6 mmol/L | 2.5–6.7 mmol/L |
| Creatinine | 56 μmol/L | 70–120 μmol/L |

The chest X-ray is shown in Fig. 21.1.

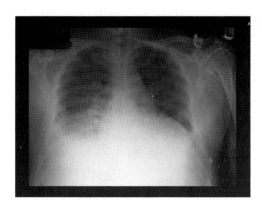

**Figure 21.1** Chest X-ray.

## Questions
- What is the diagnosis and why has it occurred?
- How would you manage this patient?

# ANSWER 21

The chest examination and X-ray suggest pulmonary oedema. Investigations show hyponatraemia and this is a recognized cause of a confusional state. There is also hypokalaemia which puts her at risk of dysrhythmia or cardiac arrest.

There has been an error in calculating the fluid deficit such that the deficit is in fact 2010 mL rather than 1010 mL. The hyponatraemia is therefore caused by fluid overload, a recognized complication of transcervical resection procedures. The normal upper limit for the procedure is 1000 mL and in this case twice that volume has been absorbed.

## Management

The mainstay of management is supportive with monitoring of electrolytes and fluid restriction. Potassium supplementation should be given and electrocardiogram (ECG) monitoring employed until the potassium is normal.

The woman should be transferred to a high-dependency bed and given oxygen. Arterial blood gas should be monitored, and if the pulmonary oedema worsens then diuretics will be needed.

The hyponatraemia usually corrects itself with time and fluid restriction, and the acute confusional state would be expected to resolve as the electrolytes normalize.

The fibroids were not completely resected and a repeat ultrasound or outpatient hysteroscopy may be considered after a few weeks to check whether further surgery is needed – sometimes degeneration may occur as a result of thermal damage or inflammation from the initial procedure. Alternatively any fibroid remnants may be expelled spontaneously through the cervix and vagina.

---

 **KEY POINTS**

- Fluid overload and consequent hyponatraemia is a recognized complication of transcervical resection procedures.
- Accurate input/output monitoring is vital during this procedure.
- Treatment is supportive until electrolytes return to normal.

---

# CASE 22: POSTMENOPAUSAL BLEEDING

## History

A 58-year-old woman reports postmenopausal bleeding for 6 months. Initially she did not pay much attention to it but she has had several episodes and it now occurs most days. It is generally light but for a few days recently it was almost like a period. There is no associated pain. The woman has never married or been sexually active. She has no previous gynaecological history and has never had a smear test. She was diagnosed with type 2 diabetes 4 years ago for which she takes oral hypoglycaemics. However she is not very compliant with diet modification, and her blood glucose is not well controlled such that starting insulin is being considered.

## Examination

The woman is obese with a body mass index of $32\,\mathrm{kg/m^2}$. Her blood pressure is 150/80 mmHg. The abdomen is non-tender, but due to her adiposity it is not possible to feel abdominal masses.

External genital examination is unremarkable. Speculum and bimanual examination are not performed as she has never been sexually active.

Transvaginal ultrasound was not possible and a transabdominal ultrasound examination was therefore performed with a full bladder.

---

 **INVESTIGATIONS**

*Transabdominal ultrasound report*: the uterus is normal size and anteverted. The endometrium could not be clearly visualized. Both ovaries appear normal. Ultrasound view was restricted by patient adiposity.

*Examination under anaesthetic and hysteroscopy*: the vagina and cervix appear normal. Hysteroscopy showed an irregular vascular mass arising from the uterine wall with contact bleeding. Curettage was performed and products sent for histological examination.

The findings at hysteroscopy are shown in Fig. 22.1.

---

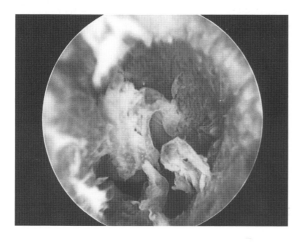

**Figure 22.1** Hysteroscopy findings. See Plate 4 for colour image.

## Questions

• What is the likely diagnosis?
• If this is confirmed how would you manage this patient?

## ANSWER 22

Postmenopausal bleeding should be considered to be due to endometrial carcinoma until proven otherwise. In many cases the diagnosis turns out to be benign. However, in this case early suspicion is raised by the risk factors for endometrial carcinoma:

- type 2 diabetes
- obesity
- nulliparity.

There is also a long history of significant bleeding suggesting a more significant pathology. In women who can tolerate the examination, the diagnosis may be made by outpatient endometrial sampling. In this case however, the inability to examine properly meant it was appropriate to investigate the uterine cavity and the rest of the lower genital tract under anaesthetic. The diagnosis of endometrial cancer was confirmed on histology report from the curettage specimen.

### Management

Management of endometrial carcinoma is simple total abdominal hysterectomy and bilateral salpingoophorectomy, as 90 per cent of women present with early-stage disease. Magnetic resonance imaging (MRI) scan prior to the procedure may be carried out to check for possible lymph node involvement, in which case lymph node biopsy should be performed at the time of surgery. Cases of stage 2 or greater disease are less common and need adjuvant radiotherapy.

Histology is needed to stage endometrial cancer:

- *stage 1*: confined to the body of the uterus
  - 1a limited to the endometrium
  - 1b invasion only of the inner half of the myometrium
  - 1c invasion to the outer half the of the myometrium
- *stage 2*: involving the uterus and cervix only
- *stage 3*: extending beyond the uterus but not beyond the true pelvis
- *stage 4*: extending beyond the true pelvis or into the bladder or rectum.

The woman should be advised that the prognosis is generally good with over 70 per cent survival at 5 years for stage 1 disease, though it is only 10 per cent for stage 4 disease.

---

 KEY POINTS

- Postmenopausal bleeding is due to endometrial cancer until proven otherwise.
- Women with prolonged or heavy bleeding are more likely to have pathology.
- Endometrial cancer is staged histologically.

---

## CASE 23: PELVIC PAIN

### History

A 24-year-old woman presents with pelvic pain and painful sexual intercourse for 2 years and is worried that she may have an ovarian cyst or other gynaecological problem. The pain occurs at any time of the menstrual cycle but is worse during menstruation. It can also be worse when she passes urine or opens her bowels. There is no relation to exercise.

She has been with her current sexual partner for 6 months and the pain occurs nearly every time she has intercourse unless penetration is very gentle. She has never been diagnosed with any sexually transmitted infections. She has been pregnant once at the age of 19 years but this ended in a spontaneous complete miscarriage.

She opens her bowels regularly and denies any bloating, constipation, diarrhoea or mucus in the stool. She had an episode of cystitis a few years ago which responded to antibiotics.

There is no other medical history of note and she takes no regular medications.

### Examination

The abdomen is not distended and there is no organomegaly. No masses are palpable but there is suprapubic tenderness. Speculum examination shows a normal smooth grey/white coloured discharge and swabs are taken. The uterus is anteverted but has limited mobility and is tender on movement. There are no adnexal masses but the adnexae are tender.

---

 **INVESTIGATIONS**

Urinalysis: protein negative; blood negative; leucocytes negative; nitrites negative

Endocervical swab: negative

Chlamydial swab: negative

High vaginal swab: negative

*Transvaginal ultrasound report*: the uterus is normal sized and axial. The endometrium measures 12 mm. Both ovaries are of normal morphology but appear adherent to the posterior uterus and show limited mobility. There is no free fluid in the pouch of Douglas.

Laparoscopy findings are shown in Figs 23.1 and 23.2.

---

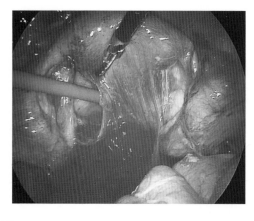

**Figure 23.1** Laparoscopy findings. See Plate 5 for colour image.

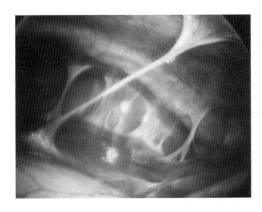

**Figure 23.2** Laparoscopy findings. See Plate 6 for colour image.

**Questions**
- What is the diagnosis?
- How would you manage this patient?
- What are the long-term implications of this disease?

# ANSWER 23

The laparoscopy image shows in Fig. 23.1 pelvic adhesions suggestive of previous infection. The 'violin-string' perihepatic adhesions in Fig. 23.2 are classical of Fitz-Hugh–Curtis syndrome, generally seen with previous chlamydial infection though also described with gonorrhoea. These findings can develop in the absence of a clinically recognized infective episode.

The woman therefore has chronic pain from pelvic inflammatory disease. Negative swabs would suggest that she may no longer be infected with chlamydia.

## Management

The pain may be helped with laparoscopic adhesiolysis. The perihepatic adhesions should be ignored as they are not causing symptoms. Otherwise pain-management options are analgesics or possible uterosacral nerve ablation.

Even though there is no evidence of current active infection, the tests have limited sensitivity so it is worthwhile treating the woman and her partner with a course of antibiotics for pelvic inflammatory disease.

---

**!** **Long-term complications of pelvic inflammatory disease**

- Chronic pain
- Infertility: tubal infertility is likely in this woman and if she fails to conceive spontaneously then hysterosalpingogram should be performed with referral for assisted conception if obstruction is confirmed
- Ectopic pregnancy: spontaneous and in vitro fertilization pregnancies are at increased risk of implanting in the damaged tubes, and an early transvaginal scan should be advised if she becomes pregnant

The woman should also be advised that despite the likely subfertility, spontaneous pregnancy may still occur so she should use effective contraception if she does not want to conceive.

---

**KEY POINTS**

- Fitz-Hugh–Curtis syndrome is the presence of perihepatic adhesions in association with previous chlamydial or gonococcal infection.
- Treatment of both partners is appropriate.
- Chronic pain, ectopic pregnancy and tubal infertility are long-term consequences of pelvic inflammatory disease.

# CASE 24: AMENORRHOEA

## History

A 14-year-old girl is seen by her general practitioner because her mother is worried that her periods have not started. Her older sister started at 13 years and her younger sister has just started her periods at 12 years, and she is now embarrassed at school as her friends are always discussing their periods and she has not told them that she has not had one.

Her mother is also concerned because she has not developed pubic and axillary hair or breast enlargement.

She was born at 38 weeks by spontaneous vaginal delivery and has never had any particular medical problems. She reached all her developmental milestones as a child although has not started a teenage growth spurt and is the second shortest girl in her class.

She eats normally with her family and denies any eating disorder. She takes part in school sport but does not exercise to excess.

She is sociable with her friends but has never had a boyfriend.

Her school academic performance is about average, although she does not do as well as her siblings who are all in the top streams of their years.

## Examination

On examination she is 120 cm and weighs 59 kg. She has no abnormal facial features but has a wide carrying angle (cubitus valgus) and a wide neck. There is no apparent breast development and the nipples appear widely spaced. No axillary hair growth is apparent.

Abdominal examination is unremarkable. The external genitalia are normal though no pubic hair is visible. Internal examination is not performed.

| INVESTIGATIONS | | |
|---|---|---|
| | | *Normal* |
| Follicle-stimulating hormone | 24 IU/L | 1–11 IU/L |
| Luteinizing hormone | 20 IU/L | 0.5–14.5 IU/L |
| Oestradiol | 84 pmol/L | 70–510 pmol/L |
| Prolactin | 239 mu/L | 90–520 mu/L |

Karyotype: 45XO

*Transabdominal ultrasound report*: the uterus appears normal size and anteverted. The endometrium appears smooth and thin, measuring 2.4 mm. Both ovaries are visualized and appear to be of small volume. No follicles are seen.

## Questions
- What is the most likely diagnosis and how might this be confirmed?
- What are the principles of management for this girl?

# ANSWER 24

The clinical features are typical of those of Turner's syndrome. This genetic condition is associated with the absence of one X chromosome (XO karyotype), occurring in approximately 1 in 2500 live female births. It is confirmed on chromosomal analysis.

In rare cases it may occurs as a mosaic form (XX/XO), in which case the features are milder and the woman may start menstruating but then experience premature ovarian failure and secondary amenorrhoea.

---

**!  Common clinical features of Turner's syndrome**

- Webbed neck
- Broad chest with widely spaced nipples ('shield chest')
- Wide carrying angle (cubitus valgus)
- Short stature (maximum 150 cm without treatment)
- Short fourth metacarpal
- Low-set ears
- Low hairline
- Hypoplastic nails
- Hypertension
- Congenital heart disease (e.g. coarctation of the aorta)

---

### Management

Management of Turner's syndrome should be carried out in a specialist referral centre.

- *Psychological*: the implications of Turner's syndrome diagnosis are devastating for the child and for the family. The absence of periods may be stigmatizing and the long-term lack of fertility is a very serious concept that may be difficult for a young girl to comprehend.
- *Medical*:
  - the short stature should be treated to enable the girl to reach her full height potential. Human growth hormone is given to achieve this.
  - oestrogen therapy initially with ethinyl estradiol enables secondary sexual characteristics of breast development and pubic and axillary hair to develop. Cyclical progestogens are added later to induce a withdrawal bleed ('period') for social reasons and to protect the endometrium from hyperplasia or malignancy in the long term. Some form of oestrogen therapy then needs to be continued until the time of natural menopause (ideally 50 years) to prevent early-onset osteoporosis in this girl.
- *Fertility*: fertility options are available with ovum donation and hormonal support.

---

**🔑  KEY POINTS**

- Turner's syndrome is a cause of primary amenorrhoea.
- Most girls will be diagnosed in early childhood because of small stature or other physical features, but some will only be diagnosed when menarche fails to occur.
- Treatment, usually hormonal, to protect bone density is essential.

---

# CASE 25: POSTCOITAL AND INTERMENSTRUAL BLEEDING

## History

A 28-year-old woman presents with intermenstrual and postcoital bleeding. She has been taking the combined oral contraceptive pill (COCP) for 4 years and has had regular light periods throughout that time. She has been with the same partner since she was 20 years and has had no previous episodes of bleeding. The bleeding is light and fresh, occurring immediately after intercourse. At other times it occurs spontaneously at unpredictable times. It varies in intensity but is never heavy. There is no associated pain.

She had a normal smear test at the age of 25 years. She has never had any sexually transmitted infections, has never been pregnant and there is no relevant previous gynaecological history.

Medically she is well and takes no medication.

## Examination

The abdomen is non-tender with no palpable masses. The external genitalia appear normal. On speculum examination the vagina appears normal as does the cervix. However, protruding through the external cervical os is a pink fleshy tumour which is freely mobile when touched with a cotton swab.

## Questions

• What are the usual differential diagnoses for irregular bleeding in women taking the COCP who have normal examination findings?
• What is the likely diagnosis in this case?
• How would you further manage this patient?

# ANSWER 25

> **!** **Differential diagnosis of irregular bleeding with the COCP, if examination is normal**
>
> - Poor compliance
> - Concurrent antibiotics (impair COCP absorption)
> - Diarrhoea or vomiting (impair absorption)
> - Infection (chlamydia, gonorrhoea or candida)
> - Cervical ectropion
> - Bleeding diathesis
> - Drug interactions (e.g. antiepileptics)

In this case the examination shows an endocervical polyp. This is generally a benign lesion that extends through the cervical canal from the endometrial cavity, on a long thin pedicle. It may be asymptomatic and found incidentally at the time of a routine smear test. Alternatively it may give rise to symptoms of intermenstrual or postcoital bleeding as in this woman.

## Management

The management is simple by avulsion in the outpatient clinic under speculum examination. The polyp is grasped with polyp forceps and twisted repeatedly until it detaches from its base. It does not matter if the whole stalk does not detach with the polyp, as any remnant generally necroses and disappears. The polyp should always be sent for histological examination although malignancy is extremely rare.

In older women or those in whom the history suggests another possible pathology, then ultrasound should be arranged to assess the endometrial cavity more thoroughly. This is not necessary in this case.

---

 KEY POINTS

- Women with irregular bleeding on the COCP should have a thorough history and examination with swabs taken for infection.
- Endocervical polyps are common and generally benign.
- Avulsion of endocervical polyps is simple in the outpatient setting.

---

# CASE 26: LABILE MOOD AND ABDOMINAL PAIN

## History

A 37-year-old mother presents to her general practitioner with cyclical labile mood swings. She says that she has always suffered with 'PMS' (premenstrual syndrome) and that it is in the family as her mother had to have a hysterectomy for the same problem. She reports her periods as always having been painful and that she has always been irritable leading up to a period. However now she feels that she is not herself for at least 2 weeks before her period and that the pain has worsened. She also notices headaches, swelling and breast tenderness.

Her periods are generally with regular bleeding for up to 6 days every 27–31 days. She has had three children all by normal vaginal delivery and the youngest is now 5 years old. She has no other medical history of note.

She has been married for 14 years and she says she often feels aggressive towards her husband or alternatively is tearful and low. Prior to having children she worked in a bank and is not sure whether to return as she feels she might be unable to cope.

## Examination

No abnormality is found on abdominal or neurological examination.

## Questions

- What is the differential diagnosis?
- How would you further determine the cause of the symptoms and manage this patient?

## ANSWER 26

The woman clearly feels that this is a gynaecological problem and that she has PMS. The diagnosis should be confirmed with evidence of symptoms occurring in the luteal phase and resolving within a day or two of menstruation starting. The differential diagnosis is depression which can manifest in a similar way to PMS.

A symptom diary is needed for recording symptoms for each day, over a 3-month period. The woman should annotate a chart with the severity of each symptom and when menstruation occurs. PMS should start after midcycle, symptoms should resolve with the period, and there should be a number of symptom-free days each month.

An example of a symptom diary is shown in Fig. 26.1.

Symptom diary

| Symptom | May | | | | | | | | | | | | | | | | | | | | | | | | | | | | | | |
|---|---|---|---|---|---|---|---|---|---|---|---|---|---|---|---|---|---|---|---|---|---|---|---|---|---|---|---|---|---|---|---|
| | 1 | 2 | 3 | 4 | 5 | 6 | 7 | 8 | 9 | 10 | 11 | 12 | 13 | 14 | 15 | 16 | 17 | 18 | 19 | 20 | 21 | 22 | 23 | 24 | 25 | 26 | 27 | 28 | 29 | 30 | 31 |
| Breast tenderness | xxx | xxx | xx | xx | xx | x | | | | | | | | | | | | | | | | | x | x | x | xx | xx | xxx | xxx | xxx | xx |
| Low mood | xxxx | xxxx | x | xxxx | xxx | xxx | x | | | | | | | | | | | | | | | | | x | xx | x | x | x | xx | xxx | |
| Feeling aggressive | xxxx | xx | xx | xxxx | xx | | | | | | | | | | | | | | | | | | | | | | x | | x | x | x |
| Bloated | x | x | xx | xx | x | x | x | | | | | | | | | | | | | | | xx | xx | xx | xxx | xxx | x | x | xx | x | xx |
| Menstruation | | | | | x | x | x | x | x | x | x | | | | | | | | | | | | | | | | | | | | |

| Symptom | June | | | | | | | | | | | | | | | | | | | | | | | | | | | | | |
|---|---|---|---|---|---|---|---|---|---|---|---|---|---|---|---|---|---|---|---|---|---|---|---|---|---|---|---|---|---|---|
| | 1 | 2 | 3 | 4 | 5 | 6 | 7 | 8 | 9 | 10 | 11 | 12 | 13 | 14 | 15 | 16 | 17 | 18 | 19 | 20 | 21 | 22 | 23 | 24 | 25 | 26 | 27 | 28 | 29 | 30 |
| Breast tenderness | x | xx | | | | | | | | | | | | | | | x | x | xx | xx | xxx | x | x | xx | xxx | xxx | xxx | xxx | x | |
| Low mood | xxx | xx | x | | | | | x | x | | | | | | | | | | | | | | | x | xx | xxx | xxx | xxx | xxx | xxx |
| Feeling aggressive | x | | | | | | | | | | | | | | | | | | x | | | x | x | | | x | x | xxx | xx | xx |
| Bloated | xx | xx | x | | | | | | | | | | | | | | | | x | | x | x | | | | x | x | xxx | xx | xx |
| Menstruation | | x | x | x | x | x | x | x | | | | | | | | | | | | | | | | | | | | | | x |

| Symptom | July | | | | | | | | | | | | | | | | | | | | | | | | | | | | | | |
|---|---|---|---|---|---|---|---|---|---|---|---|---|---|---|---|---|---|---|---|---|---|---|---|---|---|---|---|---|---|---|---|---|
| | 1 | 2 | 3 | 4 | 5 | 6 | 7 | 8 | 9 | 10 | 11 | 12 | 13 | 14 | 15 | 16 | 17 | 18 | 19 | 20 | 21 | 22 | 23 | 24 | 25 | 26 | 27 | 28 | 29 | 30 | 31 |
| Breast tenderness | | | | | | | | | | | | | | | | x | xx | xx | x | xx | xx | x | xxx | x | x | | | | | | |
| Low mood | x | | | | | | x | | | | | | | | | xxx | xxx | xxx | xxx | xxx | xxx | xxxx | xxxx | xx | xx | xx | xx | | | | |
| Feeling aggressive | x | | | | | | | | | | | | | | | | | | x | x | xx | x | x | | | | | | | | |
| Bloated | x | x | | | | | | | | | | | | | | x | xx | xx | xxx | xxx | x | x | xx | xxx | xxx | xx | xx | x | | | |
| Menstruation | x | x | x | xx | | | | | | | | | | | | | | | | | | | | | | | x | x | x | x | x |

**Figure 26.1** Premenstrual syndrome symptom diary.

### Management

If confirmed then the diagnosis should be discussed with the woman, offering appropriate understanding and support but explaining that management is variable in the success for each woman and that 'one size does not fit all'. Vitamins and oil of evening primrose are not proven in trials but may have a placebo effect.

Interruption of ovulation with the oral contraceptive pill is often successful in women under the age of 35 years.

Selective serotonin reuptake inhibitors have a good success rate in randomized trials, and the woman should be advised that they have a specific effect with PMS rather than just a general antidepressant effect.

Hysterectomy would not be helpful unless the ovaries were also removed, and this would involve risk of significant morbidity with the need for hormone-replacement therapy afterwards which may have its own side-effects or complications.

**KEY POINTS**

- Premenstrual syndrome is diagnosed with a symptom diary.
- No single treatment is effective for all women.
- Selective serotonin reuptake inhibitors are effective in many women with premenstrual syndrome.

## CASE 27: CERVICAL CANCER

### History

A 28-year-old woman was referred to the colposcopy clinic because of intermenstrual and postcoital bleeding. On examination a macroscopically visible lesion was present and on colposcopy features of malignancy were seen. Subsequent biopsy showed invasive squamous carcinoma of the cervix.

The woman was informed of the diagnosis and as a result went on to undergo an examination under anaesthetic, cystoscopy and proctoscopy for staging. The mass was found to be 3 cm in size and there was no palpable extension into the uterus, vagina or parametrial tissues. The cystoscopy and proctoscopy were both normal.

| INVESTIGATIONS | | |
|---|---|---|
| | | *Normal* |
| Haemoglobin | 12 g/dL | 11.7–15.7 g/dL |
| White cell count | $8 \times 10^9$/L | $3.5–11 \times 10^9$/L |
| Platelets | $344 \times 10^9$/L | $150–440 \times 10^9$/L |
| Sodium | 138 mmol/L | 135–145 mmol/L |
| Potassium | 3.5 mmol/L | 3.5–5 mmol/L |
| Urea | 3.6 mmol/L | 2.5–6.7 mmol/L |
| Creatinine | 76 μmol/L | 70–120 μmol/L |

*Chest X-ray report*: normal heart and lung fields. No abnormalities detected.

*Renal tract ultrasound report*: normal sized kidneys. Both ureters are of normal calibre with no evidence of obstruction.

She has had one child but had been hoping to have at least one more and is devastated by the diagnosis.

### Question

- What are the possible treatment options and their potential complications?

# ANSWER 27

Cervical cancer may be treated surgically or by radiotherapy. Staging is performed clinically at examination under anaesthetic as described.

---

**❗ Cervical cancer staging**

- *Stage 1*: carcinoma confined to the cervix
  - 1a: microscopic carcinoma
    - 1a1: stromal invasion less than 3 mm depth and 7 mm width
    - 1a2: stromal invasion up to 5 mm diameter and less than 7 mm width
  - 1b: macroscopic carcinoma
    - 1b1: up to 4 cm lesion
    - 1b2: greater than 4 cm lesion
- *Stage 2*: carcinoma extending beyond the cervix to the upper two-thirds of the vagina or parametrium
- *Stage 3*: carcinoma extending to the lower third of the vagina or the pelvic side wall
- *Stage 4*: carcinoma involves the bladder, rectum or beyond the pelvis

---

## Radical hysterectomy

Up to stage 1b women may be treated with radical hysterectomy (also known as Wertheim's hysterectomy). This involves removal of the uterus, cervix, pelvic lymph nodes and parametrial tissue as well as the upper third of the vagina. Complications involve bleeding and infection. Ureteric damage may occur and blood vessel injury is not uncommon. Postoperative complications include infections of the chest, wound or urinary tract as well as venous thromboembolism and later-onset lymphoedema from interruption of lymphatic drainage from the lower limbs.

The advantage of this treatment is that it preserves ovarian function, important for well-being and prevention of osteoporosis. It also avoids the complications of radiotherapy outlined below.

## Trachelectomy

This involves removal of the cervix, lymph nodes and parametrial tissue with conservation of the ovaries and uterine body with insertion of a suture (cerclage) at the base of the uterus. It is used selectively for women with early stage disease who wish to preserve their fertility.

## Radiotherapy

Disease beyond stage 1b, and postmenopausal women should be treated with radiotherapy which is effective but is associated with long-term effects of bowel stenosis, cystitis and vaginal stenosis. It also generally renders women menopausal due to radiation to the ovaries.

---

 **KEY POINTS**

- Cervical carcinoma should be considered in any woman with intermenstrual or postcoital bleeding.
- Disease staging is clinical, under anaesthetic.
- Cervical carcinoma may be treated surgically or by radiotherapy, depending on the stage of disease.

---

## CASE 28: URINARY INCONTINENCE

### History
A 49-year-old woman presents with leaking of urine. This started after the birth of her third child 10 years ago and has gradually worsened. She has not felt comfortable talking to her general practitioner about it until now. The leakage occurs on coughing and laughing. However she has recently started to play badminton to lose weight and the symptoms are much worse, but she has discovered though that the symptoms are much better if she wears a tampon while playing. There is no dysuria, nocturia, frequency or urgency. She is mildly constipated.

All her children were born by induction of labour post-term. They weighed 3.6 kg. 3.8 kg and 4.1 kg respectively and she needed a forceps delivery for the third child after failure to progress in the third stage. She has a regular menstrual cycle and has had a laparoscopic sterilization. There is no other relevant medical history and she takes no medications. She smokes 15 cigarettes per day and does not drink alcohol.

### Examination
Body mass index is 29 kg/m$^2$. There are no significant findings on abdominal or vaginal examination.

|  INVESTIGATIONS |
| --- |
| Urinalysis: protein negative; blood negative; leucocytes negative; nitrites negative |
| *Urodynamics report*: the first urge to void was felt at 300 mL. The maximum bladder capacity was 450 mL. Involuntary loss of urine was noted with coughing during bladder filling, in the absence of detrusor activity. |

### Questions
- What is the diagnosis?
- How would you advise and manage this woman?

# ANSWER 28

This woman is suffering from stress incontinence. Stress incontinence can be diagnosed from the history – involuntary loss of urine when the intraabdominal pressure increases (such as with exercise or coughing). Urodynamic stress incontinence (formerly referred to as genuine stress incontinence) is the involuntary loss of urine when the intravesical pressure exceeds the maximum urethral pressure in the absence of a detrusor contraction and can only be diagnosed after urodynamic testing.

## Management

### Conservative management

- Lifestyle
- The woman should be advised to control factors that exacerbate symptoms:
  - reduce weight
  - stop smoking to relieve chronic cough symptoms
  - alter diet and consider laxatives to avoid constipation
- Pelvic floor exercises: properly taught pelvic floor muscle training is a very effective treatment and can cause improvement in symptoms or cure in up to 85 per cent of women.

### Surgical management

The two main surgical techniques used currently are:

- transvaginal or transobturator vaginal tape
- colposuspension.

Both are effective but the former technique is minimally invasive and recovery is therefore more rapid. Alternative techniques such as periurethral bulking injections can be used in refractory cases or where the woman is unsuitable for surgery.

---

 **KEY POINTS**

- Stress incontinence is a clinical diagnosis.
- First-line treatment is avoidance of exacerbating factors and pelvic muscle exercises.
- Urodynamic stress incontinence should be confirmed prior to surgery.

---

## CASE 29: PELVIC PAIN

### History

A 21-year-old student presents with left iliac fossa and lower abdominal pain. The pain is present intermittently and there is no pattern to it except that it is generally worse on exercise and so she has stopped running to keep fit. The pain started about 6 months before and has gradually become more common and severe. It is no worse with her periods and she is not currently sexually active so cannot report any dyspareunia. Her periods are regular and not particularly heavy or painful. She has not had any previous gynaecological problems. She has had one sexual partner who she was with for 4 years. She denies any sexually transmitted infections.

Medically she is fit and well, and has only been admitted to hospital for wisdom teeth removal and for tonsillectomy as a child. She takes no medications.

### Examination

The woman is slim and the abdomen is soft with a palpable mass in the left iliac fossa. This is firm and feels mobile. It is moderately tender.

Speculum examination is normal. Bimanual examination confirms an 8 cm mass in the left adnexa. The uterus is palpable separately and is mobile and anteverted. The right adnexa is normal.

---

 **INVESTIGATIONS**

An abdominal X-ray is shown in Fig. 29.1.

Transvaginal ultrasound scan findings are shown in Fig. 29.2.

---

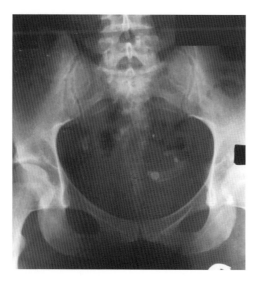

**Figure 29.1** Abdominal X-ray.

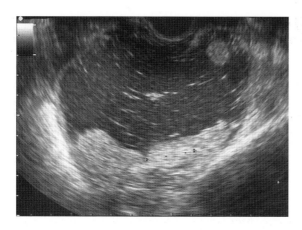

**Figure 29.2** Transvaginal ultrasound findings.

## Questions

- What is the diagnosis?
- How would you manage this woman?

# ANSWER 29

The woman has a left ovarian cyst. The ultrasound appearance shows an ovarian cyst. The appearance is of mixed echogenicity with 'acoustic shadowing' and this appearance is typical for a dermoid cyst (also known as a benign teratoma). The X-ray shows the presence of teeth in the left iliac fossa region.

These cysts are common. Typically sebaceous fluid is present, often in association with strands of hair or sometimes teeth. If active thyroid tissue develops the woman may present with features of hyperthyroidism and the cyst is referred to as a struma ovarii.

The management is surgical with ovarian cystectomy, due to the size of the cyst and the symptoms. Ideally this can be performed laparoscopically. In asymptomatic cysts there is a possibility of expectant management ('watch and wait'). However the risks of leaving the cyst are:

- malignancy occurs in up to 2 per cent of dermoid cysts
- ovarian torsion is thought to be relatively common in women with dermoid cysts and if this occurs it is a medical emergency, which may involve oophorectomy.

The woman should be advised that the cysts are common and there is very little chance that it is malignant or that removing it will affect her fertility. However, recurrence may occur in either ovary and she should seek further consultation if she develops recurrent pain.

---

  **KEY POINTS**

- Dermoid cysts (mature cystic teratoma) are a common cause of ovarian cysts in young women.
- They commonly display a classic appearance on X-ray or ultrasound scan.
- Surgery is usually recommended because of a small risk of torsion or malignant transformation.

# CASE 30: EARLY MENARCHE

## History

An 8-year-old girl is referred by the general practitioner because her periods have started. She was born at term by spontaneous vaginal delivery after an uneventful pregnancy. She has had the normal childhood illnesses but there is no significant serious medical history of note. She takes no medication. Her physical development has been unremarkable until a year ago when she changed from being average height to the second tallest in her class.

Educationally she is achieving at a similar level to her peers. She has many friends and no behavioural problems. She is the first of three children and her mother reports her own periods starting at 11 years.

## Examination

General examination is normal. The girl has significant breast bud development and some fine pubic hair. Further genital examination is not performed.

## Questions

- What is the diagnosis and what are the problems associated with it?
- How would you investigate and manage this girl?

# ANSWER 30

The average age of menarche is 13 years, and the start of periods before the age of 9 years, as in this case, is classified as precocious puberty.

In normal puberty, girls tend to start breast bud development from 9–13 years, start pubic hair growth from 10–14 years and menarche starts at 11–15 years. An increased rate of growth starts at 11–12 years and growth finishes at around 15 years. When these changes occur early but in the normal sequence, the precocious puberty is usually of no significant consequence and termed constitutional early development. This is often familial. However, if it occurs very early or in an abnormal sequence, a pathological cause is more likely

| ! Causes of precocious puberty |
| --- |
| • Constitutional (>90 per cent) |
| • Hypothyroidism |
| • CNS lesions (hydrocephaly, neurofibromatosis) |
| • Ovarian tumour |
| • Adrenal tumour |
| • Exogenous oestrogens |

## Problems of precocious puberty

- *Growth*: although the growth spurt starts early in precocious puberty, growth also stops prematurely (premature epiphyseal closure) and therefore girls with precocious puberty are at risk of having a reduced final stature if untreated.
- *Embarrassment*: early secondary sexual characteristics and the onset of periods can be very difficult for a girl to deal with at a young age.
- *Social interaction*: difficulties can occur when people who do not know the child's chronological age assume a level of intellectual and emotional maturity according to the child's physical maturity (apparent age).

## Investigation

Gonadotrophins, prolactin and thyroid hormones should be checked to confirm that they correlate with normal pubertal levels. Computerized tomography (CT) or magnetic resonance imaging (MRI) may be necessary for visualization of the pituitary stalk. Abdominopelvic ultrasound will rule out an ovarian or adrenal tumour. Bone scan will determine biological bone age to ascertain whether pituitary suppression is indicated.

## Management

As the changes in this girl seem to be in a normal sequence and she is within two years of the normal age of menarche she can be managed expectantly. However, if the changes had started at a younger age, pituitary suppression should be started with gonadotrophin-releasing hormone analogues, to delay the growth spurt and thus maintain full final height.

|  KEY POINTS |
| --- |
| • Over 90 per cent of girls with precocious puberty have constitutional (idiopathic) precocious puberty with no pathological cause, but an abnormal sequence of pubertal development or very early puberty should trigger further investigation. |
| • The major problems of precocious puberty are short final stature and social embarrassment. |

# CASE 31: EXCESSIVE HAIR GROWTH

## History

A 19-year-old woman was referred by her general practitioner (GP) with increased hair growth.

She first noticed the problem when she was about 16 years old and it has progressively worsened such that she now feels very self-conscious and will never wear a bikini or go swimming. It also affects her forming relationships. The hair growth is noticed mainly on her arms, thighs and abdomen. Hair has developed on the upper lip more recently. She has tried shaving but this seems to make the problem worse. She feels depilation creams are ineffective. Waxing is helpful but very expensive and she has bleached her upper-lip hair. Her GP has not prescribed any medication in the past.

There is no significant previous medical history of note. Her periods started at the age of 13 years and she bleeds every 30–35 days. The periods are not painful or heavy and there is no intermenstrual bleeding or discharge. She has never been sexually active.

## Examination

On examination she has an increased body mass index (BMI) of 29 kg/m². The blood pressure is 118/70 mmHg. There is excessive hair growth on the lower arms, legs and thighs and in the midline of the abdomen below the umbilicus. There is a small amount of growth on the upper lip too. The abdomen is soft and no masses are palpable. Pelvic examination is not indicated as she is a virgin.

| INVESTIGATIONS | | |
|---|---|---|
| | | *Normal* |
| Follicle-stimulating hormone (FSH) | 7 IU/L | Day 2–5 |
| | | 1–11 IU/L |
| Luteinizing hormone (LH) | 12 IU/L | Day 2–5 |
| | | 0.5–14.5 IU/L |
| Prolactin | 780 mu/L | 90–520 mu/L |
| Testosterone | 3.2 nmol/L | 0.8–3.1 nmol/L |
| Thyroid-stimulating hormone | 4.9 mu/L | 0.5–5.7 mu/L |
| Free thyroxine | 14.7 pmol/L | 10–40 pmol/L |

## Questions

- What is the likely diagnosis?
- How would you further investigate and manage this woman?

# ANSWER 31

The likely diagnosis is of polycystic ovarian syndrome (PCOS). This is supported by the clinical features of hirsutism, acne, increased BMI and slight menstrual irregularity. The biochemical results show the typical moderately raised androgen and raised LH to FSH ratio.

If the testosterone level was higher, androgen-secreting tumours should be considered (androgen-secreting ovarian, pituitary or adrenal tumours).

Other causes of hyperandrogenism include iatrogenic (glucocorticoids, danazol, testosterone), idiopathic or familial.

## Further investigation

A transabdominal ultrasound scan should be arranged to confirm the ultrasound features of polycystic ovaries, although this is not in fact an essential feature for the diagnosis of the syndrome.

## Treatment

Various treatments are used for hirsutism once serious causes of hyperandrogenism have been excluded. One of the commonest is to commence the cyproterone acetate-containing combined oral contraceptive pill (co-cyprindiol). Cyproterone acetate is an anti-androgen with progestogenic activity. It takes several months for an improvement to be seen in the hair growth and she will continue to need to use the cosmetic treatments in the meantime.

If this is ineffective then cyproterone acetate at a higher dose can be used either alone, or in addition to co-cyprindiol.

General advice should include weight loss, as this counteracts the metabolic imbalance associated with PCOS and is favourable in the long term in terms of the known cardio-vascular risks associated with hyperandrogenism.

---

 KEY POINTS

- Most women with hirsutism have PCOS or a familial tendency.
- Androgen-secreting tumours should be excluded in women with testosterone level above 5 nmol/L.
- Hirsutism has significant psychosocial consequences.

---

# EMERGENCY GYNAECOLOGY

## CASE 32: PAIN AND THE INTRAUTERINE SYSTEM

### History
A 30-year-old woman had a levonorgestrel-releasing intrauterine system (IUS) inserted by her general practitioner (GP) 3 weeks ago. Ten days ago she presented to the emergency department with abdominal pain, and on examination the threads were not visible and ultrasound scan suggested the IUS was misplaced in the right uterine cornu. An appointment was made for hysteroscopic resection but she has presented again in the interim with further pain.

### Examination
The abdomen is not distended and is soft. There is generalized lower abdominal tenderness. The threads cannot be visualized on speculum examination.

---

🔍 **INVESTIGATIONS**

*Transvaginal ultrasound report*: the uterus is anteverted and of normal size. The endometrium is regular and measures 11 mm. An IUS is not visible. Both ovaries appear normal in size and morphology.

Abdominal X-ray is shown in Fig. 32.1.

---

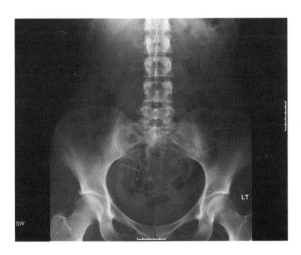

Figure 32.1 Abdominal X-ray.

### Questions
• How would you explain the symptoms and investigation findings?
• How would you further investigate and manage this patient?

# ANSWER 32

The Plain X-ray shows the IUS in the pelvis but it is lying at a transverse angle in the right pelvis. It is clearly not within the uterus. The current ultrasound result confirms that the uterus is empty. However, the previous report suggested the device was at the uterine cornu. It can be concluded therefore that the device was inserted into the uterus but it has subsequently migrated through the myometrium into the peritoneal cavity. We have no evidence to determine whether or not it was originally placed in the correct position at the fundus.

---

**!** | **Complications of intrauterine contraceptive device (IUCD)/intrauterine device insertion**

- Uterine perforation
- Device migration through to peritoneal cavity
- Pelvic inflammatory disease
- Expulsion of device (commonly with the next period)

---

### Investigation
The only important investigation is a pregnancy test, as the woman is potentially pregnant since the IUS may not have been effective if it was never in the correct location.

### Management
The IUS needs to be retrieved. While it was in the uterus this could have been performed with outpatient hysteroscopic retrieval. However, now a laparoscopy is indicated.

In this case the laparoscopy revealed blood-stained free fluid in the pouch of Douglas, with scarring on the right fundal area of the uterus. The IUS was found covered with omentum in the right lower abdomen. It was easily removed laparoscopically.

As the woman had wanted the IUS for contraception as well as treatment of her menorrhagia, and as the uterus appeared to have healed, a new IUS was inserted under laparoscopic guidance at the time. Antibiotics were given to prevent infection.

Once an IUS or IUCD has been inserted, women should be advised to have their GP check the threads are still visible after the first period. Thereafter, most women are willing and able to check the threads themselves.

---

 KEY POINTS

- The differential diagnosis of lost IUS threads is perforation and migration of the device, expulsion or misplacement of the device within the uterine cavity.
- Appropriate location at the fundus is essential for full contraceptive efficacy.
- Women with a 'lost IUCD' should use alternative contraception.

## CASE 33: BLEEDING IN PREGNANCY

### History

A 19-year-old woman presents at 13 weeks' gestation with vaginal bleeding and a smelly watery discharge. She feels generally unwell and has had fevers for the last 48 h. She initially thought she had gastroenteritis as she had reduced appetite, abdominal pain, vomited and had loose stools.

All her booking bloods were normal and the 11 week 'nuchal' scan was reassuring. She had a previous normal vaginal delivery at 38 weeks' gestation. She has no significant gynaecological or general medical history.

### Examination

On examination the temperature is 38.1°C, pulse 96/min and blood pressure 110/68 mmHg. She looks flushed and her peripheries are warm. Chest and cardiac examin-ation are normal.

She is tender over the uterus, which feels approximately 14 weeks' size. There is no guarding or rebound. On speculum examination the cervical os is closed but an offensive blood-stained discharge is seen. Bimanual examination reveals a very tender and hot uterus that also feels 'boggy'. No adnexal masses are palpable but bilateral adnexal tenderness is evident.

---

### 🔍 INVESTIGATIONS

|  |  | Normal range for pregnancy |
|---|---|---|
| Haemoglobin | 10.4 g/dL | 11–14 g/dL |
| White cell count | 24.1 × 10⁹/L | 6–16 × 10⁹/L |
| Neutrophils | 18 × 10⁹/L | 2.5–7 × 10⁹/L |
| Platelets | 556 × 10⁹/L | 150–400 × 10⁹/L |
| Sodium | 135 mmol/L | 130–140 mmol/L |
| Potassium | 3.4 mmol/L | 3.3–4.1 mmol/L |
| Urea | 6 mmol/L | 2.4–4.3 mmol/L |
| Creatinine | 80 μmol/L | 34–82 μmol/L |
| C-reactive protein | 127 mg/L | <5 mg/L |

The transvaginal ultrasound is shown in Fig. 33.1.

*Transvaginal ultrasound report*: single intrauterine gestational sac, fetus present with crown–rump length 42.7 mm, fetal heart beat absent.

---

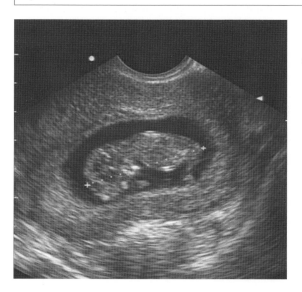

### Questions
- What is the diagnosis?
- Why is this presentation relatively uncommon in current clinical practice?
- How would you further investigate and manage this woman?

**Figure 33.1** Transvaginal ultrasound scan.

# ANSWER 33

The woman is pregnant with a dead fetus and signs of sepsis. This is referred to as a septic miscarriage. This used to be a common diagnosis due to the high incidence of illegal terminations performed by unqualified people without appropriate sterile technique, instruments or anaesthesia. Since the 1967 Abortion Act, morbidity and mortality from septic miscarriage has fallen dramatically but it remains a cause of maternal mortality, often because it is not recognized early enough. It should therefore be recognized promptly and treated aggressively.

Further investigations necessary are: blood cultures; liver function tests; coagulation screen, group and save; high vaginal and endocervical swabs.

| ! | **Complications of septic miscarriage** |
|---|---|
| | • Massive haemorrhage |
| | • Hysterectomy |
| | • Disseminated intravascular coagulopathy |
| | • Multisystem failure (secondary to haemorrhage or sepsis) |
| | • Death |

Management

- The woman should be admitted and commenced on broad-spectrum intravenous antibiotics pending culture and sensitivity.
- Aggressive intravenous fluids should be given as she has intravascular depletion due to sepsis (vasodilatation) and vomiting.
- Evacuation of retained products of conception should be arranged urgently, once the first dose of antibiotics has been given.
- A senior gynaecologist should be involved as the risks of uterine perforation or of massive haemorrhage are significant in the presence of sepsis.
- A urinary catheter should be inserted to monitor renal function.
- The woman may need transfer to the intensive care unit depending on her cardiovascular, respiratory and haematological state.

|  | KEY POINTS |
|---|---|
| | • Septic miscarriage is rare since the legalization of termination of pregnancy. |
| | • It should be recognized and treated aggressively due to the risk of rapid deterioration and mortality. |
| | • Evacuation of retained products of conception is essential to eliminate the focus of infection. |

# CASE 34: PELVIC PAIN

## History

A 27-year-old woman complains of left iliac fossa pain. The pain started while she was asleep the night before last and she says it woke her suddenly. Initially the pain was constant and severe and she was unable to get out of bed for a few hours. She felt nauseated and did not eat anything all day yesterday. There was no associated bleeding or discharge and there are no bowel or urinary symptoms. Today the pain is still present but much improved and she has been able to have breakfast.

She has had similar episodes twice in the past but they were not as severe or long-lasting. She had never been pregnant and uses the progesterone only pill (POP) for contraception. She has been with her partner for 3 years and has not had any previous sexually transmitted infections. There is no other medical history of note.

## Examination

The temperature is 37.1°C, heart rate 76/min and blood pressure 122/70 mmHg. The abdomen is slightly distended and tender in the suprapubic and left iliac fossa regions with some rebound tenderness but no guarding. No masses are palpable. Speculum examination is normal and she is tender in the left adnexa on bimanual examination, but no cervical excitation or masses are evident.

---

### 🔍 INVESTIGATIONS

|  |  | Normal |
|---|---|---|
| Haemoglobin | 12.3 g/dL | 11.7–15.7 g/dL |
| White cell count | 7.1 × 10⁹/L | 3.5–11 × 10⁹/L |
| Platelets | 402 × 10⁹/L | 150–440 × 10⁹/L |
| C-reactive protein | 2.5 mg/L | <5 mg/L |

Urinary pregnancy test: negative

Urinalysis: protein trace

Blood: negative

Leucocytes: negative

Nitrites: negative

*Transvaginal ultrasound report*: the uterus is anteverted and normal size. The endometrium is thin and measures 3.1 mm. Both ovaries appear normal. There is a moderate amount of anechoic free fluid in the pouch of Douglas, measuring 30 × 26 × 15 mm.

---

## Questions

- What is the differential diagnosis?
- How would you manage this patient?

## ANSWER 34

The sudden onset of left iliac pain suggests rupture, haemorrhage or torsion of an ovarian cyst. In cases of torsion of the ovary this would normally result in vomiting and systemic upset, whereas this woman's condition has in fact improved. In addition, an adnexal mass would be visible on ultrasound. Haemorrhage into a cyst would be seen on transvaginal ultrasound scan as an echogenic ovarian enlargement.

If a cyst ruptures then it is common for the ovary to appear ultrasonographically normal afterwards but the finding of free fluid in the pouch of Douglas suggests the former pathology.

Thus the diagnosis is likely to be a ruptured ovarian cyst. Alternative diagnoses may include irritable bowel syndrome or possibly renal colic, though urinalysis does not show haematuria.

### Management

The patient is already improving and the free fluid which is causing the peritoneal irritation (and the rebound tenderness) is expected to resolve spontaneously. Therefore immediate management is supportive with analgesia.

In the longer term, the woman should be advised to use a different contraceptive as the POP is known to be associated with an increased incidence of ovarian cysts and it seems from the history that this is the third episode for this woman.

---

 **KEY POINTS**

- The only ultrasound evidence of ovarian cyst rupture may be the presence of free peritoneal fluid.
- Ovarian cyst rupture should be managed expectantly.
- An increased incidence of ovarian cysts is found in women using the progesterone only pill, whereas the combined oral contraceptive pill reduces cyst occurrence by inhibiting ovulation.

# CASE 35: VULVAL SWELLING

### History
A 17-year-old girl presents with a vulval swelling. She noticed a lump a few weeks earlier and in the last 2 days it has enlarged and become painful. She cannot walk normally and has not been able to wear her normal jeans because of the discomfort. She feels well in herself however.

She has been sexually active since the age of 14 years and uses the depot progesterone injection for contraception and therefore does not have periods. She has been with her boyfriend for 8 months and on direct questioning reports unprotected intercourse with two other boys in that time. She had a sexual health screen in a genitourinary clinic 1 year ago and the result was normal. There is no other medical history of note and she takes no medication.

### Examination
The temperature is 37.7°C, heart rate 68/min and blood pressure normal. Abdominal examination is normal. There is a left-sided posterior labial swelling extending anteriorly from the level of the introitus, measuring $6 \times 4 \times 4$ cm. It appears red, fluctuant, tense and is exquisitely tender to touch. Bilateral tender inguinal lymph nodes are noted.

### Questions
- What is the diagnosis?
- How would you manage this patient?

# ANSWER 35

The diagnosis is of a Bartholin's abscess. The Bartholin's glands are located in the posterior vulva and the gland ducts open into the lower vagina to maintain a moist vaginal surface, important during intercourse. Obstruction to a duct by inflammation (from friction during intercourse) or infection causes a cyst to develop, which commonly becomes infected. Usually mixed flora is found but in 20 per cent of cases gonorrhoea is isolated.

The diagnosis is clinical and it is important to differentiate a Bartholin's cyst from the differential diagnosis of a sebaceous cyst, vaginal wall cyst or perianal abscess.

## Management

The abscess must be drained, traditionally by formal incision and drainage, with the edges of the cyst capsule sutured to the skin to prevent reclosure of the duct (marsupialization). Alternatively a Word catheter can be inserted for 4 weeks, which acts to allow continued abscess drainage and encourage epithelialization of the tract to provide a long-term drainage route for the gland. In most cases antibiotics are not needed after drainage, unless there is surrounding erythema or systemic signs of sepsis are present.

In this case the girl has had several recent partners and a general sexually transmitted infection screen should be arranged after drainage of the cyst, with general sexual health advice. She should also be advised that Bartholin's abscesses may recur, even after marsupialization.

---

 **KEY POINTS**

- Bartholin's abscesses are relatively common and cause acute painful unilateral vulval swelling.
- Drainage of the abscess and marsupialization of the skin edges are the mainstay of treatment but recurrence is still common.
- Pus should always be sent for culture as gonorrhoea is isolated from up to 20 per cent of Bartholin's abscesses.

---

# CASE 36: ABDOMINAL PAIN

## History

A 26-year-old woman presents with abdominal pain. It started suddenly 2 h ago and was initially in the lower abdomen but is now generalized. She feels nauseated and dizzy, especially when she sits up. She also feels as if she has bruised her shoulder. She has not noticed any vaginal bleeding or discharge, and there are no bowel or urinary symptoms.

She does not keep a record of her period dates but thinks the last one was about a month ago. She has a regular partner and says that they often forget to use a condom.

She had a termination 3 years ago. She was diagnosed with chlamydia when she was admitted to hospital at the age of 19 years with a pelvic infection.

There is no other medical history of note.

## Examination

On examination she is pale and looks unwell. She is intermittently drowsy. She is lying flat and still on the bed. The temperature is 35.9°C, pulse 120/min and blood pressure 95/50 mmHg. Peripherally she is cool and the hands are clammy. She is generally slim but the abdomen is symmetrically distended. There is generalized tenderness on light palpation, with rebound tenderness and guarding. There are no obviously palpable masses and vaginal examination has not been carried out.

Urinary pregnancy test: positive

| | INVESTIGATIONS | | |
|---|---|---|---|
| | | | *Normal* |
| | Haemoglobin | 9.6 g/dL | 11.7–15.7 g/dL |
| | Mean cell volume | 87 fL | 80–99 fL |
| | White cell count | 7.1 × 10⁹/L | 3.5–11 × 10⁹/L |
| | Platelets | 204 × 10⁹/L | 150–440 × 10⁹/L |
| | Sodium | 132 mmol/L | 135–145 mmol/L |
| | Potassium | 6.0 mmol/L | 3.5–5 mmol/L |
| | Urea | 6 mmol/L | 2.5–6.7 mmol/L |
| | Creatinine | 70 μmol/L | 70–120 μmol/L |

## Questions

• What is the likely diagnosis?
• How would you manage the patient?

# ANSWER 36

Any woman who is unwell with abdominal pain should be assumed to have a ruptured ectopic pregnancy. In this case there are risk factors and the symptoms of dizziness, nausea, severe abdominal pain and shoulder pain are classical of haemoperitoneum. The examination findings of cool and clammy peripheries, a distended abdomen, tachycardia and hypotension also suggest the clinical diagnosis and a positive pregnancy test confirms this.

Young women tend to compensate for hypovolaemia, and the fact that this woman is now cool and clammy with hypotension suggests that she is gravely unwell and should be transferred for definitive management without delay.

Although the haemoglobin does not seem dramatically reduced, it is likely that on repeat testing it may now be extremely low.

## Management

The anaesthetist, theatre staff and senior gynaecologist should be alerted immediately and the woman transferred to theatre for surgery. An ultrasound is not necessary and would increase the threat to this woman by increasing the delay in reaching theatre.

---

 **Key initial management for suspected ruptured ectopic pregnancy**

- Facial oxygen
- Lie flat with head down
- Two large-bore cannulae with 2 L of intravenous fluids given immediately
- Crossmatch 4 units (and alert haematologist to the haemorrhage)
- Consent for laparotomy and salpingectomy
- Transfer to theatre for salpingectomy

---

Ruptured ectopic pregnancy is still the leading cause of maternal death in early pregnancy, and doctors must be alert to the occasional presentation with life-threatening haemorrhage, as in this case.

---

**KEY POINTS**

- Ectopic pregnancy is still a significant cause of early-pregnancy maternal death.
- Any woman of reproductive age who is unwell with abdominal pain and a positive pregnancy test should be assumed to have a ruptured ectopic pregnancy.
- Preoperative ultrasound is not indicated if ectopic rupture is suspected.

---

# CASE 37: URINARY RETENTION

## History

A 29-year-old woman presents to the emergency department having been unable to pass urine for 8 h. For the last 3 days she has been feeling unwell with a fever, shivering and a reduced appetite. She has pain in her groins specifically but says that her whole body aches. Yesterday she began to feel pain on passing urine, and today this has became very severe such that now she cannot micturate at all. She has never experienced any episodes like this before. She has no previous medical or gynaecology history and has regular menstrual cycles. She recently ended a long-term relationship and has been with a new partner for a few months, with whom she uses condoms.

## Examination

The woman is obviously in significant discomfort. Her temperature is 37.4°C, heart rate 102/min and blood pressure 118/80 mmHg. Bilateral tender inguinal lymphadenopathy is noted and axillary lymph nodes are also palpable. The bladder is palpable midway to the umbilicus. The vulva is generally reddened and there is a cluster of ulcerated lesions of approximately 2–5 mm on the left side of the labia minora. Speculum examination shows the cervix is inflamed with a profuse exudate.

| INVESTIGATIONS | | |
|---|---|---|
| | | Normal |
| Haemoglobin | 12.7 g/dL | 11.7–15.7 g/dL |
| White cell count | 12 × 10⁹/L | 3.5–11 × 10⁹/L |
| Neutrophils | 3.2 × 10⁹/L | 2–7.5 × 10⁹/L |
| Lymphocytes | 9 × 10⁹/L | 1.3–3.5 × 10⁹/L |
| Platelets | 272 × 10⁹/L | 150–440 × 10⁹/L |

## Questions

- What is the diagnosis?
- How would you further investigate and manage this patient?

# ANSWER 37

The woman is demonstrating a classic presentation of primary herpes simplex virus infection. Prodromal 'flu type symptoms and generalized lymphadenopathy usually occur most significantly with primary infection, and any subsequent attacks are more likely to present with vulval soreness as the only noticeable feature.

---

**!  Herpes simplex features**

- *Primary infection*:
  - general malaise
  - fever
  - anorexia
  - lymphadenopathy
  - genital blisters
  - urinary retention
- *Recurrent (secondary) infection*:
  - genital blisters
  - often occurs at times of stress or tiredness

---

The woman probably acquired the infection from her new partner – condoms do not effectively prevent spread as the organism can spread from the perineum. In this case there is also evidence of herpes cervicitis from spread of virus particles into the vagina.

## Further investigation

Vulval viral swab should be sent to confirm the diagnosis. This requires firm rubbing of the swab onto an ulcer and is very painful, but as the diagnosis has such profound social implications, confirmation of the diagnosis is imperative.

## Management

- *Immediate management*:
  - the woman should have an indwelling (preferably suprapubic) urinary catheter inserted immediately and be given analgesia and paracetamol
  - local anaesthetic gel often relieves the pain and can be used until symptoms settle
  - oral aciclovir started within 24 h of an attack reduces the severity and duration of the episode.
- *Further management*:
  - referral to a health counsellor should be made to discuss the diagnosis and its implications
  - some women have many recurrent attacks, whereas others never experience a further episode. For recurrent attacks aciclovir may be given again if commenced within 24 h of becoming unwell.

---

**🔑  KEY POINTS**

- Genital herpes simplex infection has a major psychosexual and social impact on sufferers.
- The first attack is generally severe and associated with primarily systemic features.
- Recurrent episodes may be hardly noticed; transmission may occur prior to the appearance of blisters and condoms do not prevent spread of disease and so it is difficult to limit.
- Aciclovir does not cure the disease but is effective at reducing the duration and severity of an episode.

---

# CASE 38: ABDOMINAL PAIN

## History

A 14-year-old girl presents with lower abdominal pain which developed suddenly a day ago. The pain is over the whole lower abdomen but worse on the right. It was intermittent at first but is now constant and very severe. She feels unwell in herself with no appetite and vomiting. She now feels sweaty as well.

She says her bowels opened normally the day before and they are normally regular.

She has never had any previous episode of pain like this. Her last menstrual period started 2 weeks ago and she has a slightly irregular cycle. She has never had any gynaecological or other medical problems in the past.

## Examination

On examination she looks in pain and seems to find it difficult to get comfortable. Her temperature is 37.9°C, pulse 112/min and blood pressure 116/74 mmHg. She feels warm and well perfused. The abdomen is distended symmetrically with generalized tenderness, maximal in the right iliac fossa region. There is rebound and guarding in the right iliac fossa.

---

### 🔍 INVESTIGATIONS

|  |  | Normal |
|---|---|---|
| Haemoglobin | 13.8 g/dL | 11.7–15.7 g/dL |
| White cell count | $14.2 \times 10^9$/L | $3.5–11 \times 10^9$/L |
| Platelets | $390 \times 10^9$/L | $150–440 \times 10^9$/L |
| C-reactive protein | 55 mg/L | <5 mg/L |

---

## Questions

- What is the differential diagnosis?
- How would you investigate and manage this girl?

## ANSWER 38

The differential diagnosis of right iliac fossa pain in this case is:
- *gynaecological*:
  - adnexal/ovarian cyst torsion
  - ovarian cyst rupture
  - ovarian cyst haemorrhage
  - ectopic pregnancy
- *surgical*:
  - appendicitis
- *urinary*:
  - urinary tract infection
  - renal colic

The girl is acutely systemically unwell with an acute abdomen which would favour the diagnosis of torsion or possibly ruptured appendix. Cyst rupture and haemorrhage are not commonly associated with such systemic disturbance, though this is an important differential diagnosis.

Further investigation would include a pregnancy test to exclude pregnancy, and urinalysis to exclude urinary tract infection or renal colic. An ultrasound should be arranged (transabdominal) to assess for an ovarian cyst or for an inflamed appendix. If an adnexal mass is confirmed, laparoscopy or laparotomy should be performed as soon as possible since adnexal torsion is associated with loss of the ovarian function if ischaemia is prolonged and necrosis occurs. Ovarian torsion can often be managed by detorsion, though oophorectomy sometimes may be necessary.

If the diagnosis is not clear between appendicitis and ovarian torsion then joint laparotomy or laparoscopy with the surgical team is an appropriate approach.

---

 **KEY POINTS**

- Suspected ovarian torsion is a gynaecological emergency.
- Torsion is relatively common in young girls and teenagers.
- Ultrasound is useful in detection of an adnexal mass but torsion is a clinically suspected diagnosis and necessitates urgent laparoscopy or laparotomy.

## CASE 39: ABDOMINAL PAIN

### History

A 24-year-old student is referred to the gynaecologist on call from the emergency department with sudden-onset of left iliac fossa pain which woke her at 2 am. She fell asleep again but since 8 am the pain has been constant and is not relieved by ibuprofen or codydramol.

Her last period started 2 weeks ago and she reports no irregular bleeding or discharge. She has no significant gynaecological history except for a termination of pregnancy age 17 years. She has been with her current boyfriend for 2 years and has used the combined oral contraceptive pill (COCP) throughout that time. She says she has not had intercourse for the last 4 months because her boyfriend has been travelling, but says that intercourse has never been painful.

On direct questioning she has felt nauseated but has not vomited. She has had no urinary symptoms but has opened her bowels several times each day for the last 3 days, which is unusual for her.

### Examination

On examination she is apyrexial, her observations are normal and her abdomen is soft with vague left iliac fossa tenderness but no signs of peritonism. Bimanual examination reveals a normal-sized uterus with no adnexal tenderness or cervical excitation and no obvious adnexal masses.

| INVESTIGATIONS | | |
| --- | --- | --- |
| | | *Normal* |
| Haemoglobin | 12.8 g/dL | 11.7–15.7 g/dL |
| Mean cell volume | 85 fL | 80–99 fL |
| White cell count | $6.4 \times 10^9$/L | $3.5–11 \times 10^9$/L |
| Platelets | $178 \times 10^9$/L | $150–440 \times 10^9$/L |
| Sodium | 142 mmol/L | 135–145 mmol/L |
| Potassium | 3.8 mmol/L | 3.5–5 mmol/L |
| Urea | 5.0 mmol/L | 2.5–6.7 mmol/L |
| Creatinine | 72 µmol/L | 70–120 µmol/L |
| C-reactive protein | 95 mg/L | <5 mg/L |

### Questions

- What is the first investigation you would like to perform?
- What is your differential diagnosis if this test is negative, and how would you rule out some of these diagnoses?

# ANSWER 39

Any woman of reproductive age with abdominal pain should always have a urinary pregnancy test, regardless of the date of her last menstrual period. In this case the test is negative.

The remaining differential diagnoses include:

- ovarian cyst
- pelvic inflammatory disease
- urinary tract infection or stone
- bowel-related cause.

There are no specific gynaecological symptoms or adnexal tenderness, which implies that the pain is not gynaecological in origin. However, during speculum examination it is prudent to send swabs for chlamydial and gonorrhoeal infection opportunistically, in view of the high background prevalence of sexually transmitted infection, especially in the 18–25-year-old age group.

Ovulation pain (mittelschmirtz) or a corpus luteal cyst are very unlikely as the COCP inhibits the ovulatory cycle. However, a transvaginal ultrasound scan will rule out an ovarian cyst for certain.

Urine should be dipped for blood to rule out a renal stone, and for leucocytes and nitrites to rule out infection.

Bowel habit is altered and the raised C-reactive protein suggests an inflammatory condition. As the onset is acute and not severe, the diagnosis is likely to be gastroenteritis. This should be managed expectantly, with fluids, rest and simple analgesia. A stool culture should be sent if the symptoms fail to resolve. Other inflammatory bowel conditions such as Crohn's disease and ulcerative colitis are rare causes to consider if the symptoms are persistent or recurrent.

Irritable bowel syndrome is not associated with raised inflammatory markers, and is therefore not a differential diagnosis in this case.

---

 **KEY POINTS**

- Gynaecological, urinary and bowel-related pathology can all be associated with lower abdominal pain.
- A thorough and focused history is always important in making a correct diagnosis.

## CASE 40: ABDOMINAL PAIN AND VAGINAL DISCHARGE

### History

A 46-year-old Indian woman presents with a month-long history of increasing abdominal pain and a green/yellow vaginal discharge. For the last few days she had been feeling feverish and unwell. The pain is across the lower abdomen but worse on the left. She has no urinary symptoms and has been opening her bowels normally. She has a reduced appetite and mild nausea but has not vomited.

She has had two vaginal deliveries in the past and no other pregnancies. She had a laparotomy about 4 years ago for drainage of a pelvic abscess. Recently she has been under the care of a gynaecologist for heavy and prolonged periods, for which she is taking cyclical norethisterone. There is no other medical or surgical history of note.

### Examination

The temperature is 37.8°C, pulse 95/min and blood pressure is 136/76 mmHg. The abdomen appears slightly distended and a mass is palpated arising from the pelvis on the left. There is focal tenderness in the left iliac fossa without rebound tenderness or guarding. Speculum examination reveals no discharge or blood, and the cervix appears normal. Cervical excitation and bilateral adnexal tenderness are noted, more marked on the left.

---

### 🔍 INVESTIGATIONS

|  |  | *Normal* |
| --- | --- | --- |
| Haemoglobin | 10.3 g/dL | 11.7–15.7 g/dL |
| Mean cell volume | 91 fL | 80–99 fL |
| White cell count | $13.8 \times 10^9$/L | $3.5–11 \times 10^9$/L |
| Neutrophils | $8.9 \times 10^9$/L | $2–7.5 \times 10^9$/L |
| Platelets | $521 \times 10^9$/L | $150–440 \times 10^9$/L |
| C-reactive protein | 157 mg/L | <5 mg/L |

*Transvaginal ultrasound scan report*: ultrasound scan (Fig. 40.1) shows a uterus with multiple fibroids. The right ovary appears normal. The left ovary cannot be identified separately from a right adnexal complex mass, measuring $7 \times 6 \times 4$ cm.

---

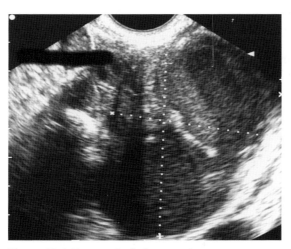

**Figure 40.1** Transvaginal ultrasound scan.

### Questions
- What is the differential diagnosis?
- Why is she anaemic?
- How would you further investigate and manage this patient?

# ANSWER 40

The woman is acutely unwell with pyrexia, tachycardia, raised inflammatory markers, neutrophilia and reactive thrombocythaemia. This suggests an infective process and the left iliac fossa mass detected on ultrasound would appear to be the cause. The likely diagnosis is a tubo-ovarian mass, probably an abscess.

Alternatively this could potentially be a diverticular abscess or, if it were on the right, an appendix abscess. Ovarian malignancy or another cause of a complex adnexal mass would be unlikely to present with this acute inflammatory episode.

Anaemia in this woman could be due to chronic menorrhagia or anaemia of chronic disease. The increased mean cell volume suggests the latter, but ferritin and folate levels would be useful to see whether there is in fact a degree of iron deficiency too.

### Further investigations
Blood cultures and vaginal and endocervical swabs should be taken. Ferritin and folate should be checked.

### Management
The woman should be admitted for intravenous antibiotics. Broad-spectrum cover should be given including agents against anaerobes and chlamydia. In cases of pelvic inflammatory disease (PID) there is commonly a mixed growth of anaerobes on top of a previous chlamydial infection. If improvement does not occur within 24–48 h, or the diagnosis is unclear, then laparoscopy or laparotomy should be performed to confirm the diagnosis and drain the abscess surgically.

---

**!**  **Advice to patients with pelvic inflammatory disease**

- The diagnosis (of PID) suggests the likelihood of a sexually transmitted infection either acutely or in the past.
- The partner needs to be screened and treated.
- The couple should avoid intercourse (or use condoms) until both have completed treatment.

---

  **KEY POINTS**

- It is common for no organism to be cultured in women with PID.
- A woman with a pelvic abscess due to PID may be given a trial of conservative treatment prior to surgical drainage.
- Contact tracing is an important part of the management of PID to prevent reinfection and further spread of infection.

# EARLY PREGNANCY

## CASE 41: BLEEDING AND PAIN IN EARLY PREGNANCY

### History
A 27-year-old woman attends the emergency department with irregular vaginal bleeding and abdominal discomfort.

She noticed the bleeding 2 days previously and it is dark red, sufficient for her to need to wear a sanitary towel, but not heavy. The abdominal discomfort is suprapubic and crampy, slightly more on the right-hand side. She is systemically well with no fever, change in appetite, nausea or vomiting. She says that her bowel and urinary habits are normal. Her last menstrual period commenced 45 days previously and she usually has a slightly irregular cycle, bleeding for 3–5 days every 28–35 days. She has never been pregnant. She has been with her regular sexual partner for 2 years and they generally use condoms but there are some occasions where they do not. She had a sexual health screen 6 months ago at the genitourinary clinic where she was told all her swabs were negative. She has no previous gynaecological history and no significant previous medical problems.

### Examination
The blood pressure is 128/72 mmHg and heart rate is 82/min. The abdomen is soft and non-distended. There is tenderness on deep palpation in the suprapubic and right iliac fossa regions, but no rebound tenderness or guarding. Bimanual examination is not performed.

| INVESTIGATIONS |
| --- |
| Urinary pregnancy test: positive |
| Transvaginal ultrasound scan is shown in Fig. 41.1. |
| The woman is taken for laparoscopy after the ultrasound scan and Fig. 41.2 shows the findings. |

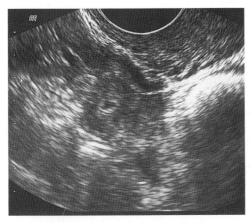

Figure 41.1 Transvaginal ultrasound scan.

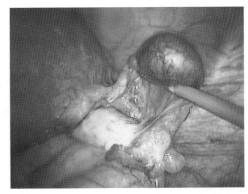

Figure 41.2 Laparoscopy findings. See Plate 7 for colour image.

### Questions
- What is the diagnosis?
- What are the management options in this case?
- How would you counsel the woman postoperatively?

# ANSWER 41

The diagnosis is an ectopic pregnancy. This can be seen from the positive pregnancy test, ultrasound confirming a pregnancy in the adnexa (with fetal heart beat present in this case), and laparoscopic confirmation of a distended right uterine tube, showing the typical bluish bulge. There is no evidence of blood in the pouch of Douglas (haemoperitoneum) to suggest rupture of the ectopic pregnancy.

Classic symptoms of ectopic pregnancy are amenorrhoea, iliac fossa pain and dark vaginal bleeding. Ectopic pregnancies are, however, often diagnosed in women with any combination of symptoms from heavy vaginal bleeding with clots to period-type pain, to no symptoms at all. Ectopic pregnancies occur in 1–2 per cent of pregnancies and the majority are diagnosed before rupture but occasionally women still present with collapse and this is a medical emergency – a woman with collapse and a positive pregnancy test should be initially assumed to have a ruptured ectopic pregnancy.

## Management options
General ectopic pregnancy management options are:

- surgical (salpingectomy or salpingotomy)
- medical (methotrexate injection)
- expectant (wait and see).

In this case, the only option is surgical in view of the fact that a fetal heart beat is present, rendering conservative options both dangerous (because of risk of rupture) and unlikely to be successful. The ectopic pregnancy should be removed laparoscopically if possible to minimize hospital stay and postoperative pain and to reduce postoperative complications including adhesions. If the contralateral tube is healthy, then the tube may be removed (salpingectomy). If the other is damaged then salpingotomy (incision into the tube to remove the pregnancy) should be attempted.

> **!** **Postoperative counselling points after ectopic pregnancy**
>
> - Explanation of diagnosis and operation
> - Appropriate counselling that the woman may grieve (this is the loss of a pregnancy) with advice about further support
> - Avoid the progesterone only contraceptive pill (POP) and intrauterine contraceptive device (IUCD) (both are associated with a slightly higher risk of ectopic pregnancy)
> - Approximately 65–70 per cent of women who have had an ectopic pregnancy go on to have a live birth following this, but there is a 10–15 per cent chance of a further ectopic pregnancy
> - Early transvaginal scan is indicated at around 5 weeks' gestation to confirm the location of any future pregnancy
> - Effective contraception should be used if she does not wish to become pregnant again at the moment

> **KEY POINTS**
>
> - The symptoms of an ectopic pregnancy are highly variable, from no symptoms to pain and bleeding, to sudden life-threatening collapse.
> - Ectopic pregnancy can only be ruled out after positive visualization of an intrauterine gestation sac.
> - 'Viable' ectopic pregnancies (where the fetal heart beat is visualized) should always be treated surgically.

# CASE 42: PAIN IN EARLY PREGNANCY

## History

A 22-year-old woman attends the emergency department complaining of abdominal pain. She is 7 weeks 4 days pregnant by certain menstrual dates. She had a normal vaginal delivery at term 18 months ago. Her periods are usually regular every 27 days, with bleeding for 3–5 days. She has no previous gynaecological history. Her medical history involves mild asthma and two episodes of cystitis.

The pain started suddenly two nights ago and is localized to the right iliac fossa with some radiation down the right thigh. It is constant though worse on movement, so she has tended to lie still. She has not taken any analgesia as she is uncertain whether this is safe for the baby. She is always constipated and this is worse since she became pregnant. She has urinary frequency but no dysuria or haematuria. She has a slightly reduced appetite but does not feel feverish or sweaty.

## Examination

Her temperature is 36.4°C, heart rate 90/min and blood pressure 96/58 mmHg. There are no signs of anaemia and she feels warm and well perfused. She is slim and the abdomen is not distended. There is focal tenderness on palpation of the right iliac fossa, with slight rebound tenderness but no guarding. Rovsing's sign is not present. Speculum examination is unremarkable. The uterus is bulky and retroverted with no cervical excitation. The right adnexa is tender with a suggestion of 'fullness'.

<table>
<tr><td colspan="3">🔍 INVESTIGATIONS</td></tr>
<tr><td></td><td></td><td>Normal range for pregnancy</td></tr>
<tr><td>Haemoglobin</td><td>12.1 g/dL</td><td>11–14 g/dL</td></tr>
<tr><td>Mean cell volume</td><td>89 fL</td><td>74.4–95.6 fL</td></tr>
<tr><td>White cell count</td><td>5.1 × 10⁹/L</td><td>6–16 × 10⁹/L</td></tr>
<tr><td>Platelets</td><td>223 × 10⁹/L</td><td>150–400 × 10⁹/L</td></tr>
<tr><td>C-reactive protein</td><td>&lt;5 mg/L</td><td>&lt;5 mg/L</td></tr>
</table>

Urinary pregnancy test: positive

Urinalysis: protein trace; blood negative; nitrites negative; leucocytes negative

Transvaginal ultrasound findings are shown in Figs 42.1 and 42.2.

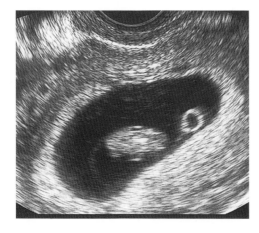

Figure 42.1 Transvaginal ultrasound scan of uterus.

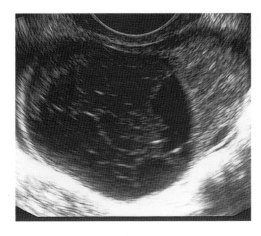

**Figure 42.2** Transvaginal ultrasound scan of right adnexa.

## Questions

- What is the likely diagnosis and what are the differential diagnoses for the pain?
- How would you further investigate and manage this woman?

# ANSWER 42

The ultrasound shows a single viable intrauterine pregnancy and haemorrhage into a corpus luteal cyst.

---

**!** **Differential diagnosis for pain in early pregnancy**

- Corpus luteum
- Ectopic pregnancy
- Miscarriage
- Ovarian cyst
- Urinary tract infection
- Renal tract calculus
- Constipation
- Appendicitis
- Unexplained pain

---

Urinary tract infection or calculi are excluded by the urinalysis result. Constipation is more likely to cause left-sided pain and the sudden onset of pain would perhaps be unusual. Appendicitis should be considered but the lack of systemic features, the normal temperature, white count and C-reactive protein are suggestive of this not being the diagnosis.

The corpus luteum is the cystic area that develops on the ovary at the ovulation site. It may be solid, cystic or haemorrhagic and may vary in size. On colour Doppler ultrasound it has a typical 'ring of fire' appearance, distinguishing it from other types of ovarian cyst. In this case the 'spider web' or reticulated pattern of echoes within the cyst suggests that it is haemorrhagic.

## Management

Management is supportive with analgesia (paracetamol in the first instance followed by codeine derivatives if necessary) and reassurance. There is no evidence that bleeding into the corpus luteum adversely affects the pregnancy outcome. As the cyst is so large, it may be sensible to repeat an ultrasound scan in 2–4 weeks to confirm resolution.

---

 **KEY POINTS**

- A large or haemorrhagic corpus luteum is a common cause of early-pregnancy pain.
- Most women have no cause found for early pregnancy pain.
- Ectopic pregnancy must be excluded and non-gynaecological aetiology considered (constipation or urinary tract infection) in women with pain in early pregnancy.

---

# CASE 43: EARLY PREGNANCY ULTRASOUND

## History

A 25-year-old woman is referred by the general practitioner (GP) for early pregnancy dating ultrasound scan. She is gravida 4 para 2. Her first positive pregnancy test was 4 days ago and she went to her GP to arrange a termination of pregnancy as she feels that she cannot cope with another child. She has been taking the combined oral contraceptive pill (COCP), so pregnancy could not be dated clinically. She has no significant gynaecological history of note except for an episode of chlamydia aged 18 years, for which she and her partner were fully treated. As a child she had a ruptured appendix and needed a midline laparotomy. She has no other relevant past medical history.

She has had no pain though did note some moderate vaginal bleeding 2 weeks before for 3 days, which settled spontaneously.

## Examination

She looks well with normal heart rate and blood pressure and a soft non-tender abdomen. Speculum examination shows a closed cervix with a normal discharge and no blood. The uterus feels normal size and is anteverted and mobile. There is no cervical excitation. There is slight tenderness in the left adnexa but no masses are palpable.

---

🔍 **INVESTIGATIONS**

Transvaginal ultrasound findings are shown in Fig. 43.1.

---

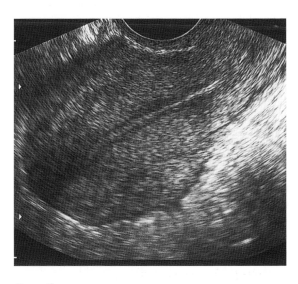

**Figure 43.1** Transvaginal ultrasound scan.

## Questions

• How would you interpret this ultrasound scan result?

Serial serum human chorionic gonadotrophin (HCG) and progesterone is requested and the results are as follows:
Day 1: serum HCG 703 IU/L, progesterone 30 nmol/L
Day 3: serum HCG 905 IU/L, progesterone 24 nmol/L

• What is the likely diagnosis and the differential diagnosis, and how would you further investigate and manage this woman?

## ANSWER 43

The transvaginal ultrasound scan shows an empty uterus and no adnexal masses. This is therefore termed a pregnancy of unknown location (PUL).

> **!** **Definition of a pregnancy of unknown location**
>
> • No signs of either intra- or extrauterine pregnancy or retained products of conception in a woman with a positive pregnancy test

PUL occurs in up to 20 per cent of women in early pregnancy units and the possible underlying diagnoses are:

- early intrauterine pregnancy: too early to be visualized on ultrasound
- failed pregnancy: a complete miscarriage where the pregnancy has been completely expelled but where no previous scan is available to confirm that an intrauterine pregnancy had been present
- ectopic pregnancy: the pregnancy is located outside the uterine cavity but has not been visualized at initial ultrasound examination.

Only 10 per cent of PULs are subsequently diagnosed as ectopic pregnancies, but all must be investigated with serial serum HCG to determine which of the above three diagnoses is likely.

### Serum HCG results and management

The HCG at which an intrauterine pregnancy would normally be visualized is 1000–1500 IU/L (in most but not all cases). A normal early pregnancy would generally show an increase in HCG of over 66 per cent in each 48 h. The progesterone level is usually high (>60 nmol/L) in an ongoing pregnancy and low (<25 nmol/L) in a failing pregnancy.

In this case the suboptimal HCG rise and mid-range progesterone are typical (but not diagnostic) of an ectopic pregnancy, and the woman should have a repeat ultrasound within a few days. If an ectopic pregnancy is visualized then medical or surgical management should depend on signs and symptoms. If a pregnancy is still not visualized and she becomes symptomatic then laparoscopy is indicated to establish the diagnosis. If HCG continues to rise with no apparent pregnancy visible, then methotrexate for persistent PUL may be considered.

>  **KEY POINTS**
>
> - Pregnancy of unknown location may represent an early intrauterine pregnancy, complete miscarriage or an ectopic pregnancy.
> - Follow-up HCG and ultrasound must be arranged for these women.
> - If pain develops before a diagnosis is confirmed, laparoscopy should be carried out to exclude an ectopic pregnancy.

# CASE 44: PREGNANCY DATING

## History

A woman is referred from the general practitioner for pregnancy dating. She had a positive pregnancy test 3 days ago after she realized that she had missed a period. In the past she had had regular cycles bleeding for 5 days every 28 days. However she had been taking the combined oral contraceptive pill (COCP) for the last 6 years and stopped only 10 weeks ago. She had a withdrawal bleed at the end of the last packet, followed by an apparently normal period 5 weeks later. She has had no other irregular bleeding or any abdominal pain. She has had regular intercourse throughout the time since she stopped her COCP and is pleased now to be pregnant.

---

 **INVESTIGATIONS**

Transvaginal ultrasound findings are shown in Fig. 44.1.

---

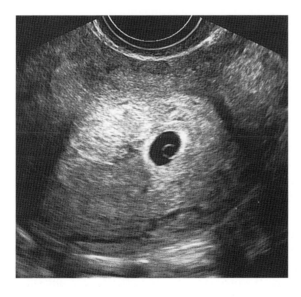

**Figure 44.1** Transvaginal ultrasound scan.

## Questions

- How can pregnancies be dated and what is the approximate gestational age for this pregnancy?
- What further investigations would you like to do to confirm this?
- Why is correct early pregnancy dating important?

## ANSWER 44

### Pregnancy dating methods

- *Dating by crown–rump length*: from 6 weeks and 2 days an estimate of gestational age can be made by crown–rump length of the fetus according to published reference values.
- *Dating by last menstrual period*:
  - in women with certain last menstrual period dates (LMP) and a regular cycle, Naegle's rule may be applied, whereby the estimated delivery date is calculated by (LMP date – 3 months) + 7 days + 1 year
  - Naegle's rule cannot be applied where the cycle is not regular or there has been a pregnancy or hormonal contraception within the last 3 months.
- *Dating by bimanual examination*: pregnancy dating by bimanual examination is very rarely performed as it is unnecessarily invasive and inaccurate.

---

**!** **Transvaginal markers in early pregnancy**

- *4–5 weeks*: appearance of gestation sac (anechoic area asymmetrically located within the endometrium towards the fundus of the uterus)
- *5 weeks*: appearance of yolk sac (a small round structure within the gestation sac supporting the fetus until the placenta develops, then disappears by 11 weeks)
- *6 weeks*: appearance of a fetal pole with a visible fetal heart pulsation within the gestation sac, separate from the yolk sac
- *7–8 weeks*: appearance of the amniotic sac, which later fuses to the chorionic membrane to become invisible on scan by 12 weeks
- *8 weeks*: appearance of fetal limb buds and fetal movements

---

The ultrasound shows an intrauterine gestation sac and a yolk sac, so in this case the pregnancy is approximately 5 weeks' gestation. This should be confirmed by re-scan (after at least 2 weeks) when a fetal pole will be visible and crown–rump length can be measured. The importance of accurate dating is:

- timing of Down's syndrome screening
- accurate gestational age estimation for cases of delivery at the borderline of viability (e.g. preterm delivery at 22–24 weeks)
- timing of induction of labour for post-term pregnancy.

---

**KEY POINTS**

- Women with uncertain LMP should be offered early first-trimester ultrasound examination to estimate gestational age.
- Standardized dating charts exist incorporating crown–rump length measurement until 14 weeks and head, femur and abdominal measurements thereafter.
- Re-scan for viability and measurement of crown–rump length is needed if the gestational sac is small and no fetus is present.

# CASE 45: PAIN AND BLEEDING IN EARLY PREGNANCY

## History

A 30-year-old woman is referred from her general practitioner. She is 11 weeks and 2 days gestation and has noticed dark spotting and mild period-like pains for the last 4 days. Her last period was 4 months ago but she has a history of polycystic ovarian syndrome and has an irregular cycle bleeding for 4–7 days every 5–6 weeks. She had a positive home pregnancy test because she noticed breast tenderness, and came for a dating ultrasound scan 4 weeks ago that confirmed a viable single intrauterine pregnancy. Since then she has had a booking visit with the midwife and all routine blood tests are normal. She is gravida 2 para 0. Her last pregnancy 9 months ago ended in a complete miscarriage at 7 weeks. There is no other medical or gynaecological history of significance.

## Examination

She is apyrexial with normal heart rate and blood pressure. The abdomen is soft and non-tender. Speculum examination shows a small cervical ectropion but this is not bleeding. The cervix is closed and no blood or abnormal discharge is seen. Bimanual examination reveals an 8–10-week-sized anteverted mobile uterus with no cervical excitation, adnexal masses or tenderness.

---

 **INVESTIGATIONS**

*Transvaginal ultrasound scan report* (Fig. 45.1): the uterus contains a gestational sac measuring 49 × 48 × 36 mm. A single fetus of crown–rump length 47 mm is visible. Fetal heart beat is absent. The uterus is anteverted. Both ovaries appear normal with no adnexal masses visible.

---

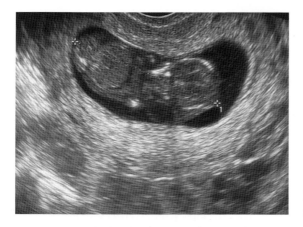

**Figure 45.1** Transvaginal ultrasound scan.

## Questions

- What is the diagnosis?
- How would you investigate and manage this patient?

# ANSWER 45

The diagnosis is of a missed miscarriage. The alternative terminology for this condition is delayed miscarriage, silent miscarriage or early fetal demise.

The diagnosis can be made for two reasons. First the fetal heart beat has been seen previously and is no longer visible. Second, where the crown–rump length exceeds 6 mm, a fetal heart beat should be visible on transvaginal ultrasound in all cases of a viable pregnancy. Thus the diagnosis could have been made even if the previous scan result was not known.

The term 'empty sac' (blighted ovum or anembyonic pregnancy) is used where the pregnancy has failed at a much earlier stage, such that the embryo did not become large enough to be visualized, but a sac is still seen. The diagnosis of an empty gestational sac can be made when the mean sac diameter exceeds 20 mm with no visible fetal pole (fetus). This is illustrated in Fig. 45.2. The management of missed miscarriage and empty sac is the same.

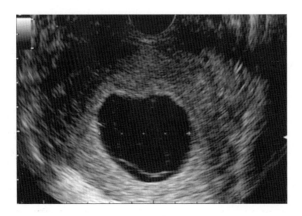

Figure 45.2 Transvaginal ultrasound image demonstrating an empty gestational sac with mean sac diameter greater than 20 mm, confirming the diagnosis of miscarriage.

## Management

The woman needs to discuss how to proceed now and also what has happened and what she might expect for future pregnancies. The management of miscarriage is expectant, medical or surgical. The choice should be given with the potential advantages and disadvantages of each:

- *expectant ('wait and see' approach):*
  - avoids medical intervention and can be managed completely at home
  - may involve significant pain and bleeding
  - unpredictable time frame – miscarriage may even take several weeks
  - more successful for incomplete miscarriage than for missed miscarriage
- *medical* (oral mifepristone followed 48h later by misoprostol intravaginal tablets):
  - avoids surgical intervention and general anaesthetic
  - the woman may retain some feeling of being in control
  - equivalent infection and bleeding rate as for surgical management (2–3 per cent)
  - surgical evacuation may be indicated if medical management fails
- *surgical* (evacuation of retained products of conception):
  - can be arranged within a few days and avoids prolonged follow-up
  - very low rate of failure (retained products of conception)
  - small risk of uterine perforation or anaesthetic complication.

Success rates for missed miscarriage are generally greater for medical or surgical management, whereas expectant management is very successful for incomplete miscarriage.

---

 **Important counselling points after miscarriage**

- Express sympathy – this is a very significant event for the couple and they may perceive the pregnancy loss as strongly as they would the loss of a full-term baby.
- Offer further counselling if needed and give written advice sheets/leaflets.
- Reassure that the miscarriage would not have been a result of anything she has done, such as lifting heavy objects, having a glass of alcohol or having sexual intercourse (all common reasons for women to feel they are responsible for the loss).
- Explain that over 60 per cent of fetal losses are due to sporadic chromosomal abnormalities such as trisomies.
- Explain that although she has had two consecutive fetal losses there is still a high chance (>70 per cent) that she will have a normal pregnancy in the future.

---

Further investigation into recurrent miscarriage is usually reserved for those with three or more consecutive losses, because miscarriage is extremely common and those couples with two miscarriages are extremely unlikely to have any underlying cause of miscarriage.

---

**KEY POINTS**

- Most miscarriages are due to sporadic fetal chromosomal abnormalities.
- A 'missed' miscarriage may be managed expectantly, medically or surgically.
- Never forget that a miscarriage may be a significant life event for a woman/couple, regardless of whether or not the pregnancy was planned.

---

# CASE 46: BLEEDING IN EARLY PREGNANCY

## History

A 36-year-old woman presents with vaginal bleeding at 8 weeks 3 days' gestation. She has never been pregnant before. Bright red 'spotting' commenced 7 days ago, which she thought was normal in early pregnancy. However since then the bleeding is now almost as heavy as a period. There are no clots. She has no abdominal pain. Systemically she has felt nausea for 3 weeks and has vomited occasionally. She had large-loop excision of the transformation zone (LLETZ) treatment after an abnormal smear 6 years ago. Since then all smears have been normal. There is no other significant gynaecological history. She has regular periods bleeding for 5 days every 28 days, and has never had any known sexually transmitted infections. In the past she used condoms for contraception.

## Examination

The heart rate is 68/min and blood pressure is 108/70 mmHg. The abdomen is soft and non-tender. Speculum reveals a normal closed cervix with a small amount of fresh blood coming from the cervical canal. Bimanually the uterus feels bulky and soft, approximately 10 weeks in size. There is no cervical excitation or adnexal tenderness.

---

**🔍 INVESTIGATIONS**

Urinary pregnancy test: positive

Figure 46.1 shows the transvaginal ultrasound findings.

---

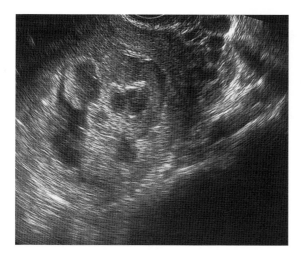

**Figure 46.1** Transvaginal ultrasound scan of the uterus.

## Questions

- What is the likely diagnosis and differential diagnosis?
- What would one expect to see at scan in this woman if the pregnancy was normal?
- How would you manage the patient?

## ANSWER 46

The ultrasound scan shows a mixed echogenicity appearance in the uterus, typical of a complete hydatidiform mole (molar pregnancy, part of the spectrum of gestational trophoblastic disease). There is no recognizable gestational sac or fetus.

This appearance may also be seen occasionally in pregnancies where early fetal demise has occurred but the sac has not been expelled (delayed miscarriage) resulting in cystic degeneration of the placenta.

The incidence of hydatidiform mole (also known as gestational trophoblastic disease) is approximately 1 in 714. It generally presents with painless vaginal bleeding though it may be diagnosed as an incidental finding when ultrasound is performed for another indication. The classical associations with hyperemesis, thyrotoxicosis or pre-eclampsia are rarely seen in the developed world where diagnosis is generally made in the first trimester.

### Normal findings at 8 weeks
The normal findings at 8 weeks would be a fetus of approximately 18 mm, with a positive fetal heart beat. The yolk sac would still be visible and the amniotic sac would also be seen. The fetus would be beginning to develop visible arm and limb buds and fetal movement may be seen.

Figure 46.2 shows a transvaginal image of a normal 8-week gestation sac and fetus.

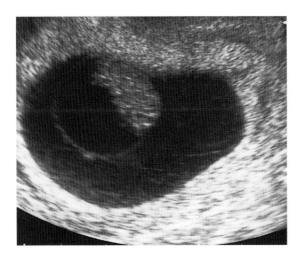

Figure 46.2 Transvaginal image of a normal 8-week gestation sac and fetus (yolk sac not visible in this view).

### Further management
The management for suspected molar pregnancy is always evacuation of retained products of conception (ERPC), with urgent histological examination of the tissue.

Once diagnosis is confirmed by histology, any woman with a confirmed partial or complete mole should be referred to a specialist gestational trophoblastic disease centre (in the UK in Sheffield, Dundee and Charing Cross Hospital) for follow-up of human chorionic gonadotrophin (HCG) levels. Women with persistently raised HCG levels are offered chemotherapy to destroy the persistent trophoblastic tissue and minimize the chance of development of choriocarcinoma.

Most women however do not require chemotherapy as the HCG becomes negative within a short period of time. These women should be advised:

- not to become pregnant again until 6 months after the HCG is normal
- there is a 1 in 84 chance of a further molar pregnancy
- they should have HCG monitoring after any subsequent pregnancy (whether live birth, fetal loss or termination)
- the combined oral contraceptive pill may safely be used once HCG has returned to normal (previous advice was to wait for 6 months).

---

 **KEY POINTS**

- Molar pregnancy may be suspected on ultrasound examination but the diagnosis must be confirmed with histological examination of products of conception after ERPC.
- Molar pregnancies must be followed up at a specialist gestational trophoblastic disease centre.
- Development of choriocarcinoma after molar pregnancy is rare, but persistent trophoblastic disease requiring chemotherapy is more common.

# CASE 47: BLEEDING IN EARLY PREGNANCY

## History

A 31-year-old woman presents with vaginal bleeding at 5 weeks 6 days' gestation. She has had a previous left uterine tubal ectopic pregnancy managed with laparoscopic salpingectomy. She is certain of her last menstrual period date and has regular cycles. Her last smear test was normal and she has not used contraception since her last pregnancy 3 years ago.

When she was 21 years she had an episode of pelvic inflammatory disease treated with intravenous antibiotics. She is otherwise not aware of having had any sexually transmitted infections. She has been with her partner for 7 years. She smokes 10 cigarettes per day and does not drink alcohol. The bleeding is described as very light and she has not been aware of any pain. She has not felt dizzy or lightheaded and has no shoulder-tip pain.

## Examination

She is warm and well perfused. The blood pressure is 136/78 mmHg and heart rate 75/min. The abdomen is not distended and no tenderness is elicited on palpation. The cervix is closed. The uterus feels normal size, anteverted and mobile, and there is no cervical excitation. Gentle adnexal examination shows no significant tenderness.

---

 **INVESTIGATIONS**

Human chorionic gonadotrophin (β-HCG): 691 IU/L

Transvaginal ultrasound scan findings are shown in Figs 47.1 and 47.2.

---

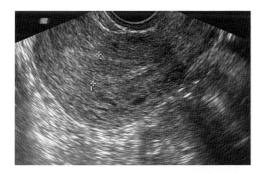

**Figure 47.1** Transvaginal ultrasound scan of the uterus.

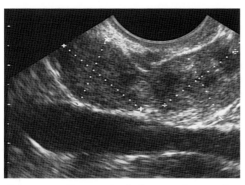

## Questions
- What is the diagnosis?
- What management options are available and which management would be preferred in this particular case?

**Figure 47.2** Transvaginal ultrasound scan of the adnexa.

# ANSWER 47

The ultrasound scan shows an empty uterus and an adnexal mass adjacent to the right ovary. The mass represents an ectopic pregnancy. No gestation sac or fetal pole is visible and the pregnancy is therefore not considered 'viable'. However there is still a possibility of rupture if not treated.

---

**!** **Risk factors for ectopic pregnancy**

- Smoking
- Previous pelvic inflammatory disease or chlamydial infection
- History of infertility
- In vitro fertilization
- Previous tubal surgery
- Previous ectopic pregnancy
- Intrauterine contraceptive device (IUCD) or progesterone only pill

---

## Management

Three options might be appropriate to this woman:

- *surgical*: laparoscopic excision of the tube (salpingectomy) or salpingotomy to incise the tube and flush out the ectopic pregnancy
- *medical*: intramuscular methotrexate to destroy the rapidly dividing trophoblast tissue, with regular HCG follow-up to confirm resolution
- *expectant*: 'wait and see' approach, suitable if the HCG at 48 h is decreasing spontaneously and the woman remains asymptomatic.

In this case the woman has previously had a uterine tube removed and surgery might compromise the remaining tube, so methotrexate treatment is preferred. However if the tube is damaged but preserved, she may be at high risk of further ectopic pregnancy. Prerequisites for methotrexate are normal full blood count, renal and liver function before treatment, compliance with the intense follow-up, and understanding the need not to become pregnant again for at least 3 months due to the potential teratogenic effects. Potential side-effects are abdominal pain (sometimes difficult to distinguish from pain suggestive of tubal rupture), nausea, diarrhoea and, rarely, conjunctivitis and stomatitis.

---

 **KEY POINTS**

- Ectopic pregnancies are commonly asymptomatic or associated with atypical symptoms.
- Surgical, medical or expectant management of ectopic pregnancy depend on the symptoms, signs and HCG result.
- Methotrexate is effective but follow-up is intensive and sometimes prolonged.

---

# CASE 48: BLEEDING IN EARLY PREGNANCY

## History

A 41-year-old woman is seen in the early pregnancy unit because of vaginal bleeding. She is gravida 4 para 2 having had two previous normal vaginal deliveries followed by a miscarriage. She has a regular 28-day menstrual cycle and her last period started 9 weeks ago. She had slight vaginal bleeding two weeks ago and on ultrasound scan an early intrauterine pregnancy had been visualized with gestational sac of $18 \times 12 \times 22$ mm diameter and a yolk sac visualized of $4 \times 5 \times 5$ mm. No fetus was visualized. She was given an appointment for a repeat ultrasound.

Four days ago her bleeding became very heavy and she passed large clots which she described as 'like liver'. She developed severe abdominal pain which lasted for about 4 h, and since then the bleeding has become very light and she is now pain free.

She has normal appetite and no nausea or vomiting. She has no urinary or bowel symptoms.

## Examination

She appears well and is apyrexial. There are no signs of anaemia. The heart rate is 82/min and blood pressure is 132/78 mmHg. The abdomen is soft and mildly tender suprapubically. Speculum shows the cervix is closed with a small amount of old blood in the vagina. There is slight uterine tenderness on bimanual palpation and the uterus feels normal size, anteverted and mobile, with no adnexal tenderness or cervical excitation.

---

| 🔍 | INVESTIGATIONS |
|---|---|
| | A transvaginal ultrasound scan is shown in Fig. 48.1. |

---

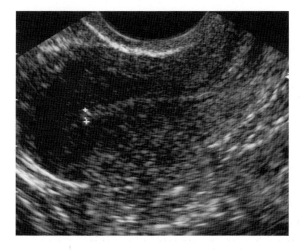

**Figure 48.1** Transvaginal ultrasound scan.

## Questions
- What is the diagnosis?
- What further management is indicated?

# ANSWER 48

The ultrasound image shows a longitudinal view of the uterus with a thin homogenous endometrium and no evidence of a gestation sac or retained products of conception. As we know from the previous report that there was previously an intrauterine pregnancy, we can conclude that this is a complete miscarriage. If a previous ultrasound had not been available we would need to treat the case as a pregnancy of unknown location and monitor serial serum HCG.

No further management is needed as the miscarriage is complete and there are no signs of retained products of conception, or any suggestion of sepsis. Anti-D is not needed even if the woman is Rhesus negative as the pregnancy is less than 12 weeks' gestation.

Counselling is the most important part of this consultation, as explained in case 45.

There is no clear evidence that a longer interpregnancy interval improves the outcome in future pregnancies, and the couple should be informed that they may try and conceive whenever they choose. However, it may be advisable to wait until after the next menstrual period (usually 4–6 weeks after a miscarriage) in order to date the pregnancy.

Reassurance scans are helpful in future pregnancies and may improve outcome. In view of the two consecutive losses, reassurance ultrasound at 7 weeks and then at intervals until the 11–14-week scan would be ideal.

---

 **KEY POINTS**

- Clinical suspicion alone is not sufficient to make a diagnosis of miscarriage.
- If the uterus is empty and an intrauterine gestation has not been previously confirmed then a case should be treated as a pregnancy of unknown location, with serial HCG follow-up.
- Appropriate counselling is vital in the management of couples with early pregnancy loss.

## CASE 49: PAIN IN EARLY PREGNANCY

### History
A 39-year-old woman presents with left iliac fossa pain in pregnancy. The pain is intermittent and cramping. She has had difficulty sleeping because of the pain, but has not taken any analgesia, as she is afraid that this may affect the baby. There is no vaginal bleeding.

The woman has a long history of secondary infertility. She had a spontaneous vaginal delivery at term 9 years ago, and started trying to conceive again soon after. She was investigated a year ago and found to have polycystic ovarian syndrome and was therefore commenced on clomifene citrate. This was her third cycle, her last menstrual period started 45 days ago and she had a positive pregnancy test 4 days ago.

### Examination
The woman is apyrexial with normal blood pressure and heart rate. She is overweight (body mass index 32 kg/m²) and therefore examination is limited but there is some tenderness on deep palpation in the left adnexa. On bimanual examination the uterus is normal size and anteverted. There is some left adnexal tenderness but no obvious masses are palpable.

---

 **INVESTIGATIONS**

Transvaginal ultrasound findings are shown in Fig. 49.1.

---

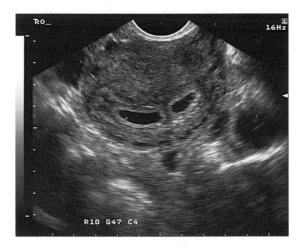

**Figure 49.1** Transvaginal ultrasound scan.

### Questions
• What can you infer about the pregnancy from this ultrasound?
• What are the differential diagnoses for the pain?
• How would you further investigate and manage this patient?

# ANSWER 49

Two distinct echolucent areas are visible within the endometrium. Each has a bright tro-phoblastic ring around confirming that these are gestation sacs. Neither sac demonstrates a definite yolk sac or fetal pole. The findings suggest a twin pregnancy with gestational age of 4–5 weeks, and this is consistent with the woman's last menstrual period date. The sacs are distinct and therefore the pregnancy will definitely be dichorionic diamniotic. Zygosity cannot be determined by this ultrasound as both dizygotic pregnancy and a monozygotic embryo that split prior to implantation would give this appearance.

Differential diagnosis of pain in this woman is:

- *gynaecological*:
  - corpus luteal cyst
  - other non-pregnancy-related incidental ovarian cyst
  - ovarian hyperstimulation (a rare complication of clomifene treatment)
- *non-gynaecological*:
  - constipation
  - gastroenteritis
  - urinary tract infection
  - renal tract calculus.

Ectopic pregnancy is ruled out as the ultrasound confirms an intrauterine pregnancy. Pelvic inflammatory disease is extremely uncommon in pregnancy as is irritable bowel syndrome.

## Further investigation

The woman should be asked about constipation or loose stools, urinary frequency, dysuria or loin pain. Urinalysis for blood (suggestive of calculus) or nitrates/leucocytes (suggest-ive of infection) should be performed with midstream urine sent for microscopy, culture and sensitivity if positive.

The adnexae should normally be examined during the ultrasound examination. A corpus luteum is a very common cause of pain in early pregnancy and shows a typical peripheral blood flow pattern resembling a 'ring of fire' on colour Doppler examination. Corpora lutea resolve spontaneously by 12 weeks' gestation.

Other ovarian cysts would also be easily seen on ultrasound – most can be safely man-aged expectantly in pregnancy unless there is a suspicion of malignancy, torsion or symp-toms are severe. Ovarian hyperstimulation is also easily recognized on ultrasound scan.

If the urinalysis is negative, there is no suggestive history of a bowel problem and the adnexae appear normal, then reassurance should be given and the patient discharged.

---

 **KEY POINTS**

- Gynaecological and non-gynaecological problems are common causes of pain in early pregnancy and should be investigated once an ectopic pregnancy has been ruled out.
- Corpus luteal cyst is probably the commonest gynaecological cause of early-pregnancy pain and is managed conservatively with analgesia and reassurance.

---

## CASE 50: VOMITING IN PREGNANCY

### History

A 28-year-old Asian woman is referred by her general practitioner (GP) with persistent vomiting at 7 weeks' gestation. She is in her second pregnancy having had a normal vaginal delivery 3 years ago. She is now vomiting up to 10 times in 24 h, and has not managed to tolerate any food for 3 days. She can only drink small amounts of water.

She saw her GP a week ago who prescribed prochlorperazine suppositories but these only helped for a few days. She feels very weak in herself and is unable to care for her son now.

On direct questioning she has upper abdominal pain that is constant, sharp and burning. She has not opened her bowels for 5 days. She is passing small amounts of dark urine infrequently but there is no dysuria or haematuria. There has been no vaginal bleeding.

There is no other medical or gynaecological history of note except that she suffered persistent vomiting in her first pregnancy requiring two overnight admissions.

### Examination

She is apyrexial. Lying blood pressure is 115/68 mmHg and standing blood pressure 98/55 mmHg. Heart rate is 96/min. The mucus membranes appear dry. Abdominal examination reveals tenderness in the epigastrium but no lower abdominal tenderness. The uterus is not palpable abdominally.

---

### 🔍 INVESTIGATIONS

|  |  | Normal range for pregnancy |
|---|---|---|
| Haemoglobin | 11.1 g/dL | 11–14 g/dL |
| Mean cell volume | 90 fL | 74.4–95 fL |
| White cell count | $8.9 \times 10^9$/L | $6–16 \times 10^9$/L |
| Platelets | $298 \times 10^9$/L | $150–400 \times 10^9$/L |
| Sodium | 131 mmol/L | 130–140 mmol/L |
| Potassium | 3.0 mmol/L | 3.3–4.1 mmol/L |
| Urea | 8.2 mmol/L | 2.4–4.3 mmol/L |
| Creatinine | 65 μmol/L | 34–82 μmol/L |
| Alanine transaminase | 30 IU/L | 6–32 IU/L |
| Alkaline phosphatase | 276 IU/L | 30–300 IU/L |
| Gamma glutamyl transaminase | 17 IU/L | 5–43 IU/L |
| Bilirubin | 12 μ/L | 3–14 μmol/L |
| Albumin | 34 g/L | 28–37 g/L |

Pregnancy test: positive

Urinalysis: protein negative; blood negative; nitrites negative; leucocytes negative; +++ ketones; glucose negative

---

### Questions
- What is the diagnosis?
- What are the potential complications of this disorder?
- How would you further investigate and manage this patient?

# ANSWER 50

The woman is suffering from hyperemesis gravidarum. This affects only less than 2 per cent of pregnancies, although more than 50 per cent of women report some nausea or vomiting when pregnant.

> **!  Definition of hyperemesis gravidarum**
>
> Severe or protracted vomiting appearing for the first time before the 20th week of pregnancy that is not associated with other coincidental conditions and is of such severity as to require the patient's admission to hospital.

> **!  Differential diagnosis of vomiting in early pregnancy**
>
> • Urinary tract infection
> • Gastroenteritis
> • Thyrotoxicosis
> • Hepatitis

The diagnosis in this case can be made because the urinalysis is negative apart from the ketones, so urinary tract infection is very unlikely. She has not opened her bowels but this is likely to be secondary to poor dietary intake and dehydration. Liver function is normal, so liver disease causing vomiting is unlikely (though abnormal liver function may occur as a result of hyperemesis itself). Thyroid function is normal, so an alternative diagnosis of hyperthyroidism causing the vomiting is unlikely.

> **!  Complications of hyperemesis gravidarum**
>
> • Wernicke's encephalopathy (from vitamin B deficiency)
> • Korsakoff's syndrome (from vitamin B, deficiency)
> • Haematemesis (from Mallory–Weiss tear)
> • Psychological – resentment towards the pregnancy and expression of desire to terminate the pregnancy

The fetus is not at risk from hyperemesis and the nutritional deficiency in the mother does not seem to affect development. The risk of miscarriage is lower in women with hyperemesis. The risk of twins and molar pregnancy has traditionally been thought to be greater in women with hyperemesis, but this is refuted in more recent research.

## Further investigation and management

Hyperemesis is a self-limiting disease and the aim of treatments is supportive, with discharge of the woman once she is tolerating food and drink and is no longer ketotic on urinalysis.

• *Fluids*: 3–4L of normal saline should be infused per day. Dextrose solutions are contraindicated as they may precipitate Wernicke's encephaolopathy and also because the woman is hyponatraemic and needs normal saline.

- *Potassium*: excessive vomiting generally leads to hypokalaemia, and potassium chloride should be administered with the normal saline according to the serum electrolyte results.
- *Anti-emetics*: first-line antiemetics include cyclizine (antihistamine), metoclopramide (dopamine anatagonist) or prochlorperazine (phenothiazine). In severe cases, ondansetron or domperidone may be effective. There is no evidence of teratogenicity in humans from any of these regimes.
- *Thiamine and folic acid*: vitamin $B_1$ (thiamine) can prevent Wernicke's encephalopathy or the irreversible Korsakoff's syndrome (amnesia, confabulation, impaired learning ability).
- *Antacids*: for epigastric pain
- *Total parenteral nutrition (TPN)*: TPN is rarely indicated but may be life saving where all other management strategies have failed.
- *Thromboembolic stockings (TEDS) and heparin*: women with hyperemesis are at risk of thrombosis from pregnancy, immobility and dehydration, and should be considered for low-molecular-weight heparin regime as well as TEDS.

## Monitoring
Daily monitoring should be carried out, with weight measurement and urinalysis for ketones and renal and liver function.

 **KEY POINTS**

- Hyperemesis gravidarum is a diagnosis of exclusion.
- There is no adverse effect on the fetus.
- Treatment is supportive.
- Thiamine replacement prevents Wernicke's encephalopathy and Korsakoff's syndrome.

# CASE 51: BLEEDING IN EARLY PREGNANCY

## History

A 23-year-old woman is referred by her general practitioner with vaginal bleeding. She noticed that there was blood on the toilet paper 2 days ago, and following this she has had bright red spotting intermittently. She has no pain and there are no urinary or bowel symptoms.

Her last menstrual period started 9 weeks and 6 days ago and she has a regular 31-day cycle. She had a positive home urine pregnancy test 3 weeks ago after she realized she had missed a period and was feeling very tired. This is her first pregnancy. She had been using condoms but with poor compliance, so the pregnancy was unplanned but she is now happy about it.

She is generally well, only having been admitted to hospital once in the past for an appendectomy at the age of 17 years. She takes no medication, does not smoke and drinks minimal alcohol. She denies any use of recreational drugs.

## Examination

The woman is apyrexial. The blood pressure is 120/65 mmHg and heart rate 78/min. The abdomen is soft and non-tender with no palpable uterus or other masses.

---

 **INVESTIGATIONS**

Transvaginal ultrasound is shown in Fig. 51.1. The crown–rump length is 25 mm (equivalent to around 9 weeks' gestation) and the fetal heart beat is seen.

---

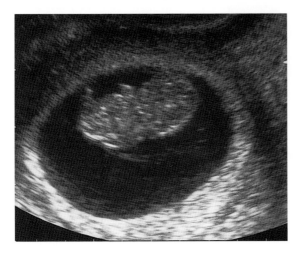

**Figure 51.1** Transvaginal ultrasound scan.

## Questions

- How would you interpret the ultrasound result?
- What further examination, investigations or management would you like to perform or request?

# ANSWER 51

The ultrasound scan shows a viable single intrauterine pregnancy. The crown–rump length is compatible with the gestational age by menstrual dates, especially as the woman reports a long menstrual cycle (3 days longer than normal, therefore gestational age would be 3 days less than the 'normal'). Where there is a significant discrepancy with menstrual and ultrasound gestational age estimation (e.g. more than 7 days), one should consider the possibility of inaccurate reporting of the last menstrual period date, irregular cycles leading to inaccurate estimated ovulation date, or of a possible growth-retarded fetus which may possibly be destined to miscarry.

In this case, as the ultrasound is reassuring the diagnosis would be of a 'threatened miscarriage'.

Figure 51.2 shows a three-dimensional image of the fetus, demonstrating the developing limbs and the physiological midgut herniation which occur at this developmental stage.

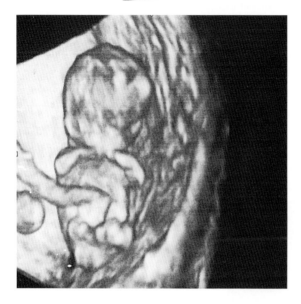

**Figure 51.2** 3D transvaginal ultrasound scan.

### Further management
A speculum examination should be performed. The possible findings may be:

- normal appearance
- cervical ectropion (often associated with postcoital bleeding)
- cervicitis (common with chlamydia)
- cervical polyp
- cervical malignancy (rare but should not be missed)
- open cervix possibly with products or clots in the os.

No further investigations are necessary at this stage – the amount of bleeding is unlikely to have caused anaemia. Rhesus status is irrelevant as anti-D immunoglobulin is only recommended with bleeding after 12 weeks' gestation, where the uterus is instrumented or where an ectopic pregnancy is treated surgically.

Management in this case is simple reassurance. Available evidence suggests that the pregnancy is at less than 5 per cent risk of miscarriage if the fetal heartbeat is normal and the bleeding resolves. There is no evidence for progesterone, bedrest or avoidance of sexual intercourse with threatened miscarriage. Further assessment should be offered if the bleeding becomes heavier or recurs. Otherwise the woman's next appointments are likely to be the antenatal midwife-booking visit and the 11–14-week ultrasound scan.

**KEY POINTS**

- Vaginal bleeding in pregnancy is associated with miscarriage in up to 50 per cent of cases, but the risk is lower if the bleeding is light.
- After a fetal heartbeat has been visualized, the chance of subsequent first-trimester miscarriage is around 5 per cent.
- Threatened miscarriage is managed by simple reassurance – there is no evidence to support the use of progesterone support, bedrest or avoidance of sexual intercourse.

# GENERAL OBSTETRICS

## CASE 52: PAIN IN PREGNANCY

### History

A 33-year-old Asian woman complains of worsening abdominal pain for 4 days. She is 16 weeks pregnant in her third pregnancy. She has a 10-year-old son, by normal delivery, and had a miscarriage 8 years ago. Her pregnancy has been uneventful until now with an unremarkable first-trimester scan.

The pain is in the left lower abdomen and is constant and sharp. She has taken paracetamol with little effect and she is unable to sleep due to the pain.

She has had no vaginal bleeding and reports urinary frequency since the beginning of the pregnancy. She is mildly constipated and has no nausea and vomiting. There is no history of trauma. She has not felt the baby moving yet.

### Examination

The woman is apyrexial and pulse rate is 125/min, with blood pressure 110/68 mmHg. The uterus is palpable just above the umbilicus. There is significant tenderness over the left uterine fundal region, where it also feels firm. The abdomen is otherwise soft and non-tender. There is voluntary guarding but no rebound tenderness. Bowel sounds are normal. Speculum examination shows a normal, closed cervix and no blood. The fetal heartbeat is heard with hand-held fetal Doppler.

| INVESTIGATIONS | | |
|---|---|---|
| | | Normal range for pregnancy |
| Haemoglobin ↓ | 10.6 g/dL | 11–14 g/dL |
| Mean cell volume | 79 fL | 74.4–95.6 fL |
| White cell count | 7.2 × 10⁹/L | 6–16 × 10⁹/L |
| Platelets | 378 × 10⁹/L | 150–400 × 10⁹/L |
| C-reactive protein | <5 mg/L | <5 mg/L |

### Questions
- What is the likely diagnosis and how should it be confirmed?
- How would you manage this woman?
- What effect will this condition have on the pregnancy?

# ANSWER 52

The diagnosis is of fibroid degeneration. The uterine size larger than dates and the localized uterine tenderness are the important features in making this diagnosis. Fibroids affect 20–30 per cent of the female population, commonly developing between 30 and 50 years. They are particularly common in African-Caribbean women.

Fibroids are oestrogen sensitive and therefore grow in pregnancy in response to the hyperoestrogenic state. When they outgrow their blood supply they undergo 'red degeneration', with necrosis within the fibroid causing the intense localized pain. The diagnosis of fibroids is confirmed by ultrasound visualization of an encapsulated mass in the uterus. The degeneration is confirmed by the ultrasound appearance of cystic spaces within the fibroid mass.

Degeneration pain usually starts gradually, and some women manage at home with simple paracetamol and rest until the pain subsides. However, it is common for the pain to be severe enough for admission to hospital for opiate analgesia. Opiates are safe in pregnancy provided use is not prolonged. Intravenous fluids may be required if the woman is not drinking, or is vomiting due to the pain.

Most women remain well systemically, although a full blood count and C-reactive protein should be taken to check haemoglobin and to assess the white blood count and inflammatory markers. In this case the woman has a mild microcytic anaemia of pregnancy and should be given ferrous sulphate.

The pregnancy itself is not usually compromised by degenerating fibroids except in the rare cases where sepsis develops, in which case miscarriage may occur.

Fibroids are managed expectantly in pregnancy but may cause malpresentation at term, or obstructed labour if there is a pelvic fibroid. In either of these circumstances, Caesarean section should be performed. Most fibroids shrink during the puerperium, so consideration of surgery should be deferred for at least 3 months after delivery.

---

 KEY POINTS

- Fibroids are common and may cause pain as they outgrow their blood supply and undergo 'red degeneration'.
- The pain is self-limiting and treatment is pain management.

# CASE 53: ILLEGAL DRUG USE IN PREGNANCY

## History

A 19-year-old woman is referred to the antenatal clinic by her general practitioner (GP). She is currently 22 weeks' gestation in her second pregnancy. She had a son by normal vaginal delivery 18 months ago, who was taken into social services care initially and now lives with his grandparents (the father's parents). Since then, the woman has been having very infrequent periods and only discovered she was pregnant when she attended the emergency department with a presumed urinary tract infection 2 weeks ago. At that stage abdominal palpation revealed a mass, and ultrasound scan confirmed the singleton gestation.

The GP letter informs that the woman has been a user of crack cocaine and heroin in the past but that she has been on a methadone replacement programme for the last 8 weeks. The current prescribed regime is 60 mL methadone, which she collects daily from the pharmacist.

The woman reports that she still injects street heroin several times per week but has not used crack cocaine for several months. She says that she drinks minimal alcohol but she smokes 20–25 cigarettes per day.

There is no other medical history of note.

She lives in a council flat with her partner who is also taking prescribed methadone. She denies any domestic violence within the relationship.

## Examination

The woman appears thin and anxious. The blood pressure is 107/65 mmHg and pulse 90/min. The abdomen is distended with the fundus palpable at the umbilicus. The fetal heartbeat is heard with a hand-held Doppler device.

| 🔍 INVESTIGATIONS |
| --- |
| Rubella: immune |
| Syphilis: negative |
| Hepatitis B surface antigen: positive |
| HIV1/2: negative |
| Haemoglobin: 11.4 g/dL |
| Blood group: A positive |

## Questions

- What other investigations should be arranged?
- What are the risks associated with drug use in pregnancy?
- How would you manage this woman during the pregnancy?

# ANSWER 53

The woman has been found to be hepatitis B surface antigen positive. This needs further investigation with e antigenicity to determine risk of transmission, and liver function tests. Assuming the hepatitis B is related to needle sharing, she is also at significant risk of hepatitis C and this should also be tested for at this stage.

A urine toxicology screen should be performed with the woman's consent, to confirm the drug history she has given and what the risks to the fetus may be.

---

**!** **Illegal drug use risks**

- *Crack cocaine*: crack cocaine use is associated with placental abruption and hence increased risk of perinatal death or prematurity. It is also known to cause intrauterine growth restriction by way of arterial vasoconstriction.
- *Heroin*: opiates are not teratogenic but are associated with intrauterine growth restriction and premature delivery.
- *Cannabis*: cannabis is not known to have specific risks in pregnancy, but the tobacco use associated and the possibility of other associated drug use makes it an important risk factor.
- *Tobacco*: tobacco use is associated with fetal growth restriction and low birth weight. There is also the risk of respiratory disease in the infant from passive smoking.

---

## Management of the pregnancy
### Multidisciplinary team

Most units have a specialist team for management of drug-using women in pregnancy. This should include specialists in substance misuse, a social worker, a specialist midwife and an interested obstetrician.

### Opiate replacement

The woman needs to be encouraged to engage more fully with the methadone replacement programme. This may well mean increasing the methadone regime to allow her to stop the street heroin. Once this has been achieved then she can gradually reduce the dose needed, with appropriate support. It is better to be still taking a maintenance dose of methadone through the pregnancy than to try and stop too quickly, resulting in unquantifiable amounts of illegal drugs being taken during the pregnancy.

### Fetal monitoring

The fetus should be assessed for growth during the pregnancy in view of the increased risk of intrauterine growth restriction.

### Delivery

Labour should be managed as for any non-drug-using woman. The difference may be that the usual doses of opiates needed for analgesia (epidural or systemic) may be insufficient and need to be titrated up to ensure adequate pain control.

Fetal blood sampling should be avoided in labour due to the risk of vertical transmission of hepatitis B antigen.

### Postpartum

The baby should be administered hepatitis B immunoglobulin at delivery and be given the accelerated hepatitis B immunization course.

Babies of opiate-using mothers may have initial respiratory depression as a result of the opiates but then develop withdrawal symptoms. They need immediate transfer to the neonatal unit for management of the symptoms, with reducing doses of opiates.

Issues of care for the baby should be established between the social services, medical team and the parents, prior to delivery.

 **KEY POINTS**

- Women who use illegal drugs have high-risk pregnancies.
- A team approach that encourages trust and engagement from the woman is likely to be most effective.
- Fetal growth should be monitored and the fetus transferred to the neonatal unit at delivery for management of respiratory depression and withdrawal.

# CASE 54: ANTENATAL SCREENING

## History

A woman aged 23 years is referred by her general practitioner to the antenatal clinic at 14 weeks in her first pregnancy. She has booked late having only just discovered she is pregnant. Although the pregnancy was unplanned she is now happy about it. She separated from her partner of 2 years a few weeks ago but is supported by her family and friends. She has no significant medical history and is one of four siblings. On direct questioning her mother apparently had a stillbirth attributed to some form of congenital abnormality 28 years ago. Otherwise the pregnancy is assessed to be low risk.

As she is too late for a nuchal translucency test she is offered serum screening for Down's syndrome, which she agrees to. This is performed at 17 weeks.

 **INVESTIGATIONS**

Alpha-fetoprotein (AFP): 3.36 multiples of the median (MoM)

Oestriol: 1.08 MoM

Human chorionic gonadotrophin (HCG): 0.89 MoM

## Questions

- How should she be counselled and what further options are available?
- If the pregnancy is not affected with a fetal abnormality, how else could this test result be explained?

# ANSWER 54

AFP, oestriol and β-HCG are used in combination in the 'triple test', one of the serum-screening tests available to detect Down's syndrome. The results are expressed as multiples of the median (MoM) and in this case the AFP is significantly raised.

Down's syndrome is associated with decreased AFP, increased oestriol and increased β-HCG.

Increased AFP is associated with an increased risk of fetal abnormality, the commonest being:

- neural tube defects
- anterior abdominal wall defects
- Patau's syndrome (trisomy 13).

The woman should be counselled that the risk of Down's syndrome is low but that the blood test suggests a possible increased risk of the other abnormalities described.

She should be referred to a specialist fetal medicine centre for a detailed ultrasound scan to exclude any significant neural tube or abdominal wall defects. Depending on the ultrasound result, she may wish to terminate the pregnancy if a serious abnormality is detected, or to continue but with appropriate geneticist and paediatric input antenatally to prepare for the delivery.

One of the problems with serum screening is that other pregnancy complications may lead to a higher level of AFP. These include:

- multiple pregnancy
- fetal intrauterine growth restriction
- oligohydramnios.

AFP is also affected by ethnic background, maternal diabetes and maternal liver disease. Finally the normal range is dependent on gestation, and unless the gestational age has been confirmed, the AFP may be high because the pregnancy is more advanced than presumed.

---

 **KEY POINTS**

- Maternal AFP is raised in the presence of neural tube defects and other fetal genetic and structural abnormalities. In contrast it is reduced in cases of Down's syndrome.
- Women with raised AFP should have their gestation confirmed by ultrasound and be referred for specialist fetal medicine ultrasound assessment for abnormalities.

# CASE 55: EPILEPSY IN PREGNANCY

## History

A 24-year-old woman attends for pre-pregnancy counselling. Her general practitioner (GP) referral letter is shown.

*Dear Doctor*

*Please could you see and advise this young woman who wishes to start a family in the near future?*

*She was diagnosed with grand mal epilepsy when she was 12 and has been on medication since then. She was initially under a paediatric neurologist but for the last 6 years has been under my care at the practice. Her current treatment regime includes sodium valproate, phenytoin and lamotrigine. She last had a fit around 1 month ago.*

*She recently married and is keen to start a family as soon as possible. I would be grateful if you could see her to discuss the management of any pregnancy. She has never been pregnant before.*

*Yours sincerely*

## Questions

- What specific risks are there in pregnancy for this woman?
- How should she be managed?

# ANSWER 55

The incidence of epilepsy in women of child-bearing age is approximately 1 in 150.

The risks of epilepsy in pregnancy can be divided into risks to the mother and to the fetus.

## Risks to the mother

Increased plasma volume causes reduced drug levels and a possible increase in fits. Other causes of increased fit frequency include excessive tiredness and hyperemesis. Some women also decide to stop their medication because of fears of adverse effects on the baby, although this may actually increase the risk to the baby as a result of a higher likelihood of prolonged fits.

## Risks to the fetus

There is an increased risk of congenital abnormality due to antiepileptic drugs (7 per cent risk for one drug, with risk increasing with multiple drugs). The risk probably applies similarly to all antiepileptic medications used.

There is also an intrinsic increased risk of epilepsy in the offspring of an epileptic mother, and during the pregnancy the fetus is also at risk of fetal hypoxia from uncontrolled maternal epilepsy.

## Management principles

### Pre-pregnancy

- Refer for neurology opinion and minimize the number of drugs, aiming for a single drug regime.
- If no fits have occurred for at least 2 years consider stopping all medication.
- Advise the woman to continue her medication during pregnancy, as having an increased number of fits is likely to increase the risk of fetal hypoxia.
- Prescribe preconceptual folic acid (5 mg daily rather than 400 µg) to minimize the risk of neural tube defects and prevent folate deficiency seen with antiepileptic regimes.

### Antenatal

- Plan for joint medical and obstetric care.
- Monitor plasma levels of anticonvulsant regime (levels are likely to diminish due to increased plasma volume).
- Advise the woman to take showers instead of baths to minimize the risk of drowning if a fit occurs in the bath.
- Arrange detailed anomaly scan and a fetal echocardiography at around 18–20 weeks for cardiac abnormalities.
- Start vitamin K from 36 weeks' gestation, to correct any potential clotting deficiency from the inhibition of clotting factor production by anticonvulsants and thus reduce the chance of fetal bleeding (e.g. intraventricular haemorrhage). The baby should also receive intramuscular (rather than oral) vitamin K at birth.
- There are no specific differences in labour management from non-epileptic women.

### Postnatal

- Anticonvulsant therapy is not a contraindication to breast-feeding.
- Decrease medication doses as maternal physiology returns to normal.
- Adequate social support is vital and plans need to be made for safe care of the infant (due to the risk of fits in the mother).

**KEY POINTS**

- Pre-pregnancy fits should be well controlled, aiming for a single drug regime.
- Epileptic medication is associated with an increased risk of congenital abnormality but the risk to the mother and baby of stopping medication usually takes priority over the risk of fetal abnormality.
- Drug compliance during pregnancy must be emphasized.

## CASE 56: BLEEDING IN PREGNANCY

### History

A woman presents at 20 weeks' gestation reporting vaginal bleeding. The bleeding occurred 2 h ago and was bright red. She reported no abdominal pain with the bleeding and she had not had any previous episodes. She had had intercourse the previous evening.

Her last cervical smear was normal 2 years ago.

This is her first pregnancy and her current obstetric history is unremarkable with normal first-trimester scan and Down's syndrome screening. She reports that her booking blood tests had been normal.

She is extremely anxious when seen, concerned that she is going to have a miscarriage.

### Examination

The blood pressure is 105/65 mmHg and pulse 86/min. Abdominal examination confirms that the uterus reaches to 1 cm below the umbilicus. The uterus is soft and non-tender. The fetal heart is heard with the hand-held fetal Doppler ultrasound probe. Speculum examination reveals a reddened area around the external cervical os, with an inflammatory appearance and a small amount of contact bleeding. The os itself is closed.

### Questions
- What is the most likely cause of the bleeding?
- How would you manage this woman?

# ANSWER 56

One of the commonest causes of bleeding in pregnancy is a cervical ectropion, and this is suggested in this case by the examination findings. An ectropion can often look florid and inflamed even in the absence of infection.

An ectropion may occur at any time in a woman's reproductive life but tends to be prevalent:

- in pregnancy
- after puberty
- with the combined oral contraceptive pill.

Postcoital bleeding often suggests an ectropion or other cervicitis. However, caution should be exerted as an ectropion is very common in pregnancy and could be an incidental finding when there is in fact a uterine source of bleeding. Thus the findings in this case are very suggestive of bleeding secondary to an ectropion but do not fully rule out a uterine source of the blood loss.

The woman should generally be reassured about the likely cause of the loss. She should be given anti-D if Rhesus negative, as a fetomaternal haemorrhage could potentially have occurred if this was uterine bleeding.

Swabs should be taken during the speculum examination to rule out chlamydia, as well as microscopy, culture and sensitivity for organisms including group B streptococcus and candida.

Above the gestational age of fetal viability (23–24 weeks), a woman would normally be admitted for observation for possible further bleeding and risk of premature delivery. However at 20 weeks with no possibility of fetal viability, there is no advantage to admission to hospital with light bleeding.

Bedrest has not been shown to be of benefit in cases of vaginal bleeding in pregnancy.

She should be advised that the ectropion is not harmful to the pregnancy but may result in further bleeding episodes, in which case she should be seen again in the obstetric department.

---

 **KEY POINTS**

- Women with bleeding in pregnancy must have a speculum examination.
- Swabs should be taken at the time of speculum examination.
- After 23 weeks the woman should be admitted if bleeding continues, due to the risk of premature delivery.

# CASE 57: GLUCOSE TOLERANCE TEST

## History

A woman attends the antenatal day assessment unit to discuss the result of her glucose tolerance test. She is 42 years old and this is her sixth pregnancy. She has previously had three Caesarean sections, one early miscarriage and a termination of pregnancy. All booking tests were normal as were her 11–14-week and anomaly ultrasound scans.

The woman is of Indian ethnic origin but was born and has always lived in the UK. She is now 26 weeks' gestation and her midwife arranged a glucose tolerance test because of a family history of type 2 diabetes (her father and paternal aunt).

## Examination

The body mass index (BMI) is 31 kg/m². Blood pressure is 146/87 mmHg. The symphysiofundal height is 29 cm and the fetal heart rate is normal on auscultation.

| INVESTIGATIONS |
| --- |
| Urinalysis: 1+ glycosuria |
| Glucose tolerance test (75 g glucose drink): <br> pretest fasting blood glucose: 6.4 mmol/L; <br> 2 h blood glucose following 75 g oral glucose load: 11.3 mmol/L. |

## Questions
• What is the diagnosis and on what criteria can this be made?
• What are the principles of management for this patient?

# ANSWER 57

The diagnosis is of gestational diabetes mellitus (GDM) and is based on the 2 h glucose concentration exceeding 11.1 mmol/L (World Health Organization (WHO) criteria). The diagnosis may also be made if the fasting blood glucose exceeds 7.8 mmol/L, in which case a formal glucose tolerance test would not have been necessary. Transient glycosuria is common in pregnancy and may occur after a glucose-rich drink or snack. Therefore the urinalysis alone is unhelpful in the assessment of this woman.

GDM occurs in up to 3 per cent of the pregnant population depending on the ethnic diversity of the specific population. In some cases it may be the first presentation of previously undiagnosed diabetes.

---

**!  Risk factors for GDM**

- *Pre-existing*:
  - obesity
  - previous GDM
  - family history of diabetes
  - women with previously large babies or stillbirth
  - increasing maternal age
- *Occurring in this pregnancy*:
  - glycosuria
  - large for dates baby
  - polyhydramnios

---

The importance of the diagnosis relates to the effect on the mother and fetus.

- *Effects on the fetus*:
  - fetal macrosomia
  - polyhydramnios
  - neonatal hypoglycaemia
  - neonatal respiratory distress syndrome
  - increased stillbirth rate
- *Effects on the mother*:
  - increased risk of traumatic delivery (e.g. shoulder dystocia)
  - increased Caesarean section risk
  - increased risk of developing GDM in subsequent pregnancies
  - 50 per cent increased risk of developing type 2 diabetes within 15 years

## Management principles
- Optimal control of maternal blood glucose minimizes the chance of fetal complications. This needs the multidisciplinary input of a diabetologist, specialist diabetes nurse, dietitian, specialist midwife and obstetrician.
- Dietary advice and counselling are the initial interventions (reduced fat and carbohydrate intake with weight control).
- Blood glucose monitoring at home should be initiated with pre- and post-prandial levels at each meal.
- Oral hypoglycaemics are contraindicated in pregnancy.
- If blood glucose measurements are repeatedly high, insulin should be commenced.

- The fetus should be monitored with regular ultrasound scans for growth and liquor volume (polyhydramnios being a sign of fetal polyuria secondary to excessive glucose level).
- Delivery should be planned by 40 weeks, but Caesarean section should be performed for obstetric indications only.
- Sliding-scale insulin should be initiated in labour for women on insulin.
- The insulin can be stopped immediately postpartum as normal glucose homeostasis returns rapidly after delivery.
- The fetus should be carefully monitored for neonatal hypoglycaemia.
- The mother should have a repeat glucose tolerance test 6 weeks postpartum to rule out pre-existing diabetes.

 **KEY POINTS**

- Gestational diabetes should initially be treated with dietary and weight advice. Insulin may be needed if blood glucose levels remain high.
- One-third of women with impaired glucose tolerance in pregnancy will go on to develop diabetes mellitus in the next 25 years.

# CASE 58: ANTENATAL SCREENING

## History

A woman aged 34 years is 9 weeks' gestation in her third pregnancy. Her first pregnancy ended in a first-trimester suction termination at 18 years of age and she had a miscarriage 8 months ago requiring evacuation of retained products of conception (ERPC). She is generally well except for mild asthma.

She has no family history of congenital abnormalities. She is a non-smoker and currently drinks approximately 3 units of alcohol per week. Her only medication is folic acid 400 µg daily.

Her partner is 31 years old and was adopted. He has no known medical problems.

The routine booking blood and urine tests are normal. The couple opt for Down's syndrome screening and a first-trimester ultrasound appointment is booked for 12 weeks.

---

 **INVESTIGATIONS**

The first-trimester ultrasound findings are shown in Fig. 58.1.

*Ultrasound report*:

Single fetus. Fetal heart action normal

Crown–rump length 62.4 mm (corresponds to 12 + 3 weeks' gestation)

Nuchal translucency (NT) 3.2 mm

Risk of trisomy by maternal age (34 years) 1:276

Adjusted risk of trisomy after NT 1:30

---

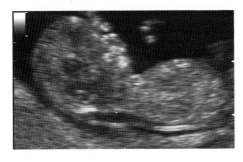

**Figure 58.1** First trimester ultrasound scan.

## Questions

- How would you explain the report to the couple?
- What are the options available to the couple now and what are their relative advantages and disadvantages?
- The couple chose to have a further test and the results are normal, what further diagnoses should be considered?

# ANSWER 58

### Explanation of the report

Down's syndrome screening can be difficult to explain, and any discussion should start with checking that the couple understand what Down's syndrome is:

- a chromosomal 'genetic' problem that usually occurs sporadically ('by chance')
- associated with physical abnormalities which may be relatively minor, such as short stature, abnormal facial appearance, or major, such as severe cardiac abnormality
- always associated with learning disability, though the extent is variable
- life expectancy is generally up to 40 or 50 years.

The 'nuchal translucency' test is a screening test and does not give a definite answer as to whether the pregnancy is affected or not. The risk in this case based on the mother's age alone is 1 in 276, but the high NT measurement combined with the maternal age suggests that the risk for this particular baby is 1 in 30. Most women even with a high risk result actually have a normal fetus (a false-positive result).

### Available options

Any risk above 1 in 250 to 300 is considered 'high risk' and such women are offered diagnostic testing to give a definite diagnosis. Samples are obtained by chorionic villous sampling (CVS) at 11–14 weeks or by amniocentesis from 15 weeks. Both involve an ultrasound-guided needle inserted through the abdominal wall under local anaesthetic. Both are associated with approximately 1 in 100 risk of procedure-related miscarriage. CVS can be performed earlier, which allows for earlier termination if that is chosen, but has a risk of not giving a true result (mosaicism). Amniocentesis is performed from 15 weeks and has no risk of placental mosaicism.

A couple may alternatively choose to avoid invasive testing and have a detailed anomaly scan at 20 weeks to assess for 'soft markers' of Down's syndrome (such as skull abnormalities, ventriculomegaly, atrial septal defect, duodenal atresia, echogenic bowel, hydronephrosis and short limbs).

This couple opts for amniocentesis at 16 weeks' gestation and the result is:

- *Chromosomal analysis: 46XY normal karyotype.*

### Further investigation

Fetuses with a high-risk NT but normal karyotype have an increased likelihood of other structural defects such as congenital heart disease, exomphalos, diaphragmatic hernia and skeletal defects. This couple should therefore have a detailed anomaly scan and fetal cardiac echo at around 20 weeks' gestation.

---

 **KEY POINTS**

- Nuchal translucency (NT) is a screening test not a diagnostic test.
- The NT result may increase their risk but most women with increased NT have a normal fetus (false positive). However women who have a high-risk NT and normal karyotype are at risk of other structural defects, so a detailed anomaly scan should be performed at around 20 weeks.

---

# CASE 59: ANTENATAL CARE

## History

A woman attends a routine antenatal appointment at 31 weeks' gestation. She is 26 years old and this is her fourth pregnancy. She has three children, all spontaneous vaginal deliveries at term. Her third child is 18 months old and the delivery was complicated by a post-partum haemorrhage (PPH) requiring a 4 unit blood transfusion. This pregnancy has been uncomplicated to date, with normal booking blood tests, normal 11–14-week ultrasound and normal anomaly ultrasound scan.

She feels generally tired and attributes this to caring for her three young children. She reports good fetal movements (more than 10 per day).

## Examination

Blood pressure is 126/73 mmHg.

---

**INVESTIGATIONS (blood tests taken at 28 weeks)**

| | | *Normal range for pregnancy* |
|---|---|---|
| Haemoglobin | 7.8 g/dL | 11–14 g/dL |
| Mean cell volume | 68 fL | 74.4–95.6 fL |
| White cell count | $11.2 \times 10^9$/L | $6–16 \times 10^9$/L |
| Platelets | $237 \times 10^9$/L | $150–400 \times 10^9$/L |

Urinalysis: negative

Blood group: A negative

No atypical antibodies detected.

---

## Questions

- What is the likely diagnosis and what are the implications for the pregnancy?
- What further investigations would you wish to arrange?
- How will you manage this woman for the last trimester of pregnancy?

## ANSWER 59

The haemoglobin is significantly low even for pregnancy, and is associated with a low mean cell volume. This is usually due to iron-deficiency anaemia. Iron deficiency anaemia usually occurs when the woman enters pregnancy with depleted iron stores, although she may not at that stage have low haemoglobin or any signs or symptoms suggestive of anaemia.

---

**!** **Implications of anaemia in pregnancy**

- *Baby (possible)*:
  - low birth weight
  - neonatal anaemia
  - cognitive impairment
- *Mother*:
  - antenatal
    - fatigue
    - fainting
    - dizziness
  - peripartum
    - increased risk of haemodynamic compromise
    - increased likelihood of transfusion

---

At delivery, blood loss is inevitable. This woman has additional risk factors of having her fourth delivery and having a history of PPH. As she is already very anaemic, she may decompensate easily if blood loss occurs, increasing her likelihood of hypovolaemic shock and need for emergency blood transfusion.

### Further investigations

Although the likely cause of these indices is iron deficiency, differential diagnoses include a mixed folate and iron deficiency, thalassaemia, chronic bleeding, or anaemia of chronic disease (e.g. renal disease). A full history should therefore be taken to exclude chronic diseases and to elicit any family history of thalassaemia.

Iron deficiency should be demonstrated with findings of low mean cell haemoglobin (MCH) and low serum ferritin. Ferritin below 12 μg/L confirms the diagnosis. Serum and red cell folate should also be checked and the woman should be screened for haemoglobinopathies.

If chronic disease is suspected, then further investigations may be indicated such as renal and liver function tests for chronic disease, or gastrointestinal tract endoscopy for causes of chronic bleeding.

### Further management

#### Correction of anaemia

- The woman should be prescribed ferrous sulphate 200 mg twice daily, increasing to three times if tolerated. If iron tablets are not tolerated then alternatives include iron suspension or parenteral (intramuscular) iron injections. These are painful and do not increase the serum haemoglobin more than the maximum expected from oral iron (1 g/dL per week).
- In extreme cases, where it is not possible to increase the haemoglobin level by iron supplementation, blood transfusion should be considered.
- An iron-rich diet should be encouraged.

*Delivery*

- At delivery, she should be considered at high risk of PPH and have an intravenous cannula inserted in labour, with full blood count and group and save.
- Active management of the third stage is essential (syntometrine, controlled cord traction) and an oxytocin infusion considered if bleeding is excessive or the uterus is suspected to be atonic.
- Following delivery, the woman should continue iron supplementation until iron stores (ferritin) are restored, even if haemoglobin is normal.

 **KEY POINTS**

- Anaemia (not physiological) must be investigated in pregnancy.
- If untreated, anaemia will worsen during pregnancy and blood loss at delivery may be catastrophic.
- Women with previous PPH must have active management of the third stage.

# CASE 60: PREVIOUS CAESAREAN SECTION

## History

A woman is referred to the obstetric antenatal clinic by the community midwife after the booking appointment revealed that she had had a previous emergency Caesarean. You are the foundation year 2 doctor seeing her and you elicit the history and examine her.

She is 25 years old and pregnant with her second child. Her daughter was born 3 years ago by emergency Caesarean section for failure to progress in labour due to an occipito-posterior position. The pregnancy had been uncomplicated and she had gone into spontaneous labour at 40 weeks 5 days. She had contractions for 24 h, and during this time she underwent artificial rupture of membranes and was given a syntocinon infusion for 8 h. The cervix dilated to 8 cm but she did not progress further despite regular strong contractions.

Following the emergency Caesarean the baby was well, but the woman was readmitted to hospital after 7 days because of an infected wound haematoma for which she required intravenous antibiotics.

The antibiotics altered the taste of the breast milk and the baby subsequently had to have formula milk.

She now feels anxious that she might have to go through the same experiences again and is wondering whether she can request an elective Caesarean section to avoid having another long labour and emergency procedure, with its associated complications.

She has had no other pregnancies and is generally fit and healthy. She is currently 16 weeks' gestation and has had a normal nuchal scan. Booking blood tests are normal.

## Examination

The abdomen is distended, compatible with pregnancy. The low transverse scar is visible and is non-tender. The uterus is palpable to midway between the symphysis pubis and the umbilicus. The fetal heartbeat is heard with a hand-held Doppler machine.

## Question
• How should you advise and manage her?

# ANSWER 60

The current average Caesarean section rate in the UK is approximately 24 per cent. This means that many women are returning in subsequent pregnancies having had a previous Caesarean section. In this case the woman has an otherwise low-risk pregnancy and the only factor to be considered at this stage is the planned mode of delivery.

She should be able to make an informed choice after appropriate information regarding vaginal birth after Caesarean section versus planned Caesarean section.

The important points for this woman to be informed about and to consider are summarized:

- *vaginal birth after Caesarean (VBAC)*:
  - successful in 70 per cent of cases
  - emergency Caesarean section rate is approximately 30 per cent
  - 1 in 200 risk of uterine rupture (scar dehiscence)
  - close cardiotocograph monitoring is needed, with intravenous access, fasting and full blood count and group and save serum available
  - normal progress is expected and augmentation of labour is not usually recommended in women with a uterine scar
  - induction of labour may be appropriate in selected women with previous Caesarean section
- *planned Caesarean section*:
  - operative delivery is associated with higher risks of haemorrhage, infection, visceral damage and thrombosis
  - mobility and ability to care for child and baby is more impaired by Caesarean section than vaginal delivery
  - planned Caesarean does avoid the possibility of an emergency procedure
  - after two Caesarean sections a further Caesarean would be the only option in any subsequent pregnancy

The woman should be offered a further appointment towards the end of the third trimester to confirm her decision regarding mode of delivery and to check for any complications that might contraindicate vaginal delivery such as breech presentation, a large baby, scar tenderness or pre-eclampsia. One of the most important points in the consultation is to listen to her concerns about the previous delivery and what her fears might be. An empathetic approach will help her to feel confident about any decision she makes this time.

---

 **KEY POINTS**

- Although low, the maternal morbidity and mortality are higher for Caesarean section than for vaginal delivery.
- The chances of a successful vaginal delivery after a previous Caesarean section are >70 per cent
- A woman's experiences of previous deliveries are very important in counselling for any subsequent pregnancy and delivery.

## CASE 61: GROUP B STREPTOCOCCUS

### History

You are asked to see a woman in the antenatal assessment unit. She is gravida 4, para 1, having had a normal vaginal delivery 3 years ago, a first-trimester miscarriage and two first-trimester terminations.

She is currently 26 weeks' gestation. One week ago she was seen because she experienced vaginal bleeding. At the time a small cervical ectropion had been noticed and as the bleed had occurred postcoitally, it was assumed likely to be secondary to the ectropion.

However, as per protocol, she had vaginal and endocervical swabs sent and a full blood count and group and save sample requested.

---

🔍 **INVESTIGATIONS**

|  |  | Normal range for pregnancy |
|---|---|---|
| Haemoglobin | 10.1 g/dL | 11–14 g/dL |
| Mean cell volume | 76 fL | 74.4–95.6 fL |
| White cell count | $8.0 \times 10^9$/L | $6–16 \times 10^9$/L |
| Platelets | $183 \times 10^9$/L | $150–400 \times 10^9$/L |

Blood group: A positive

No atypical antibodies detected

Endocervical swab: chlamydia negative, gonorrhoea negative

High vaginal swab: candida – small numbers identified

Group B streptococcus: positive culture.

---

### Questions
- How would you interpret these results?
- How would you manage the pregnancy and delivery in light of these results?

# ANSWER 61

The key results are

- mild anaemia
- group B streptococcus carrier
- candida.

The anaemia is mild for pregnancy and as the mean cell volume is low, suggesting iron deficiency, it may be treated with ferrous sulphate 200 mg twice daily, with repeat haemoglobin after 4 weeks. She should also be advised about an appropriate iron-rich diet (e.g. meat, lentils, spinach).

Candida organisms are present very commonly in the vagina, particularly in pregnancy. This should be treated (with vaginal clotrimoxazole) only if the woman is symptomatic (itching or lumpy discharge).

### Group B streptococcus (GBS)

GBS (*Streptococcus agalactiae*) colonization occurs in 25 per cent of women at some stage during their pregnancy. In this case the finding of GBS may relate to the presenting symptom of bleeding, but is most likely to be an incidental finding. This is the most important result as there is a risk of GBS to the baby with an incidence of 1 in 2000 neonates being infected, with 6 per cent mortality.

---

**!  Babies at particular risk of GBS infection**

- Previous baby affected by GBS
- GBS in the vagina or urine at any stage during the current pregnancy
- Preterm delivery
- Prolonged rupture of membranes
- Pyrexia in labour

---

In the UK, universal screening for GBS has not been shown to be effective in reducing neonatal death.

### Management

Antenatal treatment does not seem to reduce the neonatal risk (perhaps because of recolonization). However measures are taken to reduce transmission to the baby *at the time of delivery*:

- intravenous penicillin (or clindamycin or erythromycin if allergic) should always be given to the mother in labour
- neonatal care depends on the clinical scenario but may include:
  - observation of the baby for up to 5 days postpartum for signs of sepsis
  - consideration of culture of the baby for evidence of infection (ear, nose, axilla)
  - intravenous antibiotics until culture results confirm no evidence of infection.

---

**KEY POINTS**

- GBS is the most common cause of serious bacterial infection in UK infants, with a mortality of 10 per cent.
- Antenatal treatment is not effective but treatment instead at the time of delivery reduces perinatal morbidity and mortality.

---

# CASE 62: TWIN PREGNANCY

## History

A 37-year-old woman attends the antenatal clinic at 18 weeks' gestation. She is gravida 2 para 1, having had a spontaneous vaginal delivery at term 8 years ago. This current pregnancy was achieved through in vitro fertilization after four attempts (cycles). Two embryos were implanted. The first-trimester scan confirmed a twin gestation and noted a lambda sign between the gestations sacs. The anomaly scan is due in 2 weeks.

So far the woman has been feeling nauseated and tired but well.

## Examination

The blood pressure is 120/78 mmHg. The fundus is palpable 2 cm above the umbilicus. Two separate fetal hearts are heard on hand-held fetal Doppler, one 143/min, the other 130/min.

---

### 🔍 INVESTIGATIONS

|  |  | Normal range for pregnancy |
|---|---|---|
| Haemoglobin | 9.8 g/dL | 11–14 g/dL |
| Mean cell volume | 71 fL | 74.4–95.6 fL |
| White cell count | $5.3 \times 10^9$/L | $6–16 \times 10^9$/L |
| Platelets | $204 \times 10^9$/L | $100–400 \times 10^9$/L |

Urinalysis: negative

Haemoglobin electrophoresis: sickle trait (AS)

Blood group: A positive

Rubella antibody: immune

HIV1/2: negative

Hepatitis B: negative

Syphilis: negative

*12-week transabdominal ultrasound scan report*: two viable fetuses present, measuring 82 mm and 80 mm.

---

## Questions

- How would you interpret the results?
- What can the parents be told about the zygosity of the pregnancy?
- How would you monitor and manage this pregnancy?

# ANSWER 62

The ultrasound confirms a twin pregnancy with a lambda sign (projection of placental tissue between the dividing membranes). This is suggestive of a dichorionic pregnancy. The woman is anaemic with a low mean cell volume suggestive of iron-deficiency anaemia. The only other investigation of note is that the woman has sickle trait.

## Zygosity

Although the pregnancy appears dichorionic diamniotic (DCDA), this does not inform us about zygosity. A monozygotic pregnancy may be DCDA if the embryo has split at an early stage. One third of monozygotic pregnancies are DCDA, two-thirds monochorionic diamniotic and around 1 per cent are monochorionic monoamniotic. Confirmation of zygosity is with placental histology, or by observing that the fetuses are of different genders.

## Monitoring

Twin pregnancies are associated with increased maternal risks of hyperemesis, anaemia, preterm labour, antepartum haemorrhage, pre-eclampsia, gestational diabetes, thrombosis and Caesarean delivery.

The fetuses are at risk of intrauterine growth restriction, prematurity, stillbirth or neonatal death, congenital anomalies and operative delivery.

> **!** | **Monitoring in twin pregnancies**
>
> - Regular full blood count
> - Close blood pressure and urinalysis monitoring
> - Fetal growth surveillance from 28 weeks
> - Screening for gestational diabetes

## Management

In addition to routine antenatal care this woman needs:

- information regarding the increased maternal and fetal risks with twin pregnancy
- regular hospital antenatal assessment from the late second trimester
- ferrous sulphate and folic acid supplementation
- discussion of mode of delivery (depending on growth and presentation of twins at around 36 weeks)
- hospital delivery by 40 weeks
- introduction to multiple pregnancy support groups.

The woman has sickle trait and her partner should also be tested. If he is also sickle trait positive then prenatal testing of the babies should be offered to determine whether they are homozygous and therefore going to be affected by sickle cell disease.

> **KEY POINTS**
>
> - Chorionicity and amnionicity can be determined with high accuracy by ultrasound in the first trimester but, unless the fetuses are seen to be of different sexes, the zygosity of dichorionic diamniotic twins can only be confirmed with genetic or histological testing.
> - Multiple pregnancies are high risk for both mother and babies, and close monitoring is essential for the early detection of problems.
> - A woman with sickle cell trait whose partner is also sickle cell trait positive should be offered prenatal diagnosis by chorionic villus sampling, amniocentesis or cordocentesis.

# CASE 63: POSTPARTUM PYREXIA

## History

A 29-year-old woman presents with a fever. She had a Caesarean section 3 weeks ago and was recovering well until 2 days ago when she became very cold and shivery at night. She has been unable to keep herself warm despite several blankets and has reduced appetite, nausea, vomiting and lethargy. She is breast-feeding and has had very sore nipples since the birth but feels this is normal and has been using camomile ointment to soothe them. In the last 24 h she has noticed the left breast has become sore and red.

She has mild lower abdominal pain at the site of the Caesarean section wound. She no longer has vaginal bleeding but has a moderate brown discharge with an odour which she says is improving. Bowel habit is normal and she has no urinary symptoms.

## Examination

On examination the woman is wearing a jersey and jacket, with a blanket over her. Her temperature is 38.6°C. Blood pressure is 120/64 mmHg and heart rate 106/min. The chest is clear and heart sounds are normal. The right breast is normal but there is a well-demarcated area of redness over the superiolateral aspect of the left breast, which is tender and hot to touch.

The uterus is firm and is non-tender, just palpable above the symphysis pubis. There is no leg swelling.

| INVESTIGATIONS | | |
|---|---|---|
| | | *Normal range for pregnancy* |
| Haemoglobin | 10.1 g/dL | 11–14 g/dL |
| White cell count | 23.2 × 10⁹/L | 6–16 × 10⁹/L |
| Neutrophils | 19 × 10⁹/L | 2.5–7 × 10⁹/L |
| Platelets | 457 × 10⁹/L | 150–400 × 10⁹/L |
| C-reactive protein | 203 mg/L | <5 mg/L |
| Sodium | 137 mmol/L | 130–140 mmol/L |
| Potassium | 3.9 mmol/L | 3.3–4.1 mmol/L |
| Urea | 9 mmol/L | 2.4–4.3 mmol/L |
| Creatinine | 78 μmol/L | 34–82 μmol/L |

Urinalysis: +++ blood; protein trace; leucocytes negative; nitrites negative.

## Questions

- How would you interpret the investigations?
- What is the likely diagnosis and differential diagnosis?
- How would you investigate and manage this woman?

# ANSWER 63

The blood and protein on urinalysis are likely to be due to contamination from persisting vaginal discharge (lochia), but there is no evidence of urinary tract infection (no leucocytes or nitrites).

The haemoglobin is slightly low, which can occur with sepsis but is also common after pregnancy and delivery. The leucocytosis with neutrophilia and raised C-reactive protein suggests a significant bacterial septic process. Urea is raised while creatinine and potassium are normal, suggesting dehydration secondary to sepsis, pyrexia and vomiting.

## Diagnosis

The diagnosis is mastitis (a localized infection within the breast tissue). This occurs in 5 per cent of lactating women. The pathophysiology probably involves colonization of the breast ducts by bacteria through the cracked nipples, causing localized inflammation and obstruction of the duct with subsequent retention of milk, and infection. The commonest organism is staphylococcus from the skin. The differential diagnosis is of a breast abscess which would be palpated as a fluctuant mass in the breast.

## Investigation

Blood cultures and a swab from the breast milk or nipple are necessary. In cases of diagnostic doubt, an ultrasound scan can differentiate mastitis from an abscess.

## Management

The woman should be admitted for intravenous antibiotics and fluids, regular paracetamol, analgesia and anti-emetics as necessary. Until cultures are available, flucloxacillin should be commenced with consultation with a microbiologist if some improvement is not seen within 24 h.

She should be encouraged to continue breast-feeding. If this is too painful she should express milk in order to try to unblock the duct. If an abscess is diagnosed then needle aspiration under local anaesthetic is preferred to formal incision and drainage in most cases.

---

 **KEY POINTS**

- Mastitis is a common cause of puerperal pyrexia.
- As well as antibiotics, management includes continued breast-feeding from both breasts or expressing milk to unblock the duct.

## CASE 64: BLEEDING IN PREGNANCY

### History
You are asked to review a nulliparous woman who has presented with vaginal bleeding at 39 weeks + 5 days' gestation. Booking blood pressure was 123/72 mmHg. Her last midwife visit was 10 days ago when blood pressure was 130/76 mmHg.

This evening she noticed a small 'gush' of blood and discovered a bright red stain in her underclothes. She denies actual abdominal pain but reports some intermittent lower abdominal discomfort. The baby has been moving normally during the day.

### Examination
She is warm and well perfused. Her blood pressure is 158/87 mmHg and heart rate 84/min. The symphysiofundal height is 36 cm and the fetus is cephalic with 3/5 palpable abdominally. Moderate uterine tenderness is noted. The uterus is soft but during the palpation two moderate uterine tightenings are noted. On speculum examination the cervical os is closed and there is a moderate amount of vaginal blood.

---

🔍 **INVESTIGATIONS**

Urinalysis: + protein; ++ blood; leucocytes negative; nitrites negative

The cardiotocograph (CTG) is shown in Fig. 64.1.

---

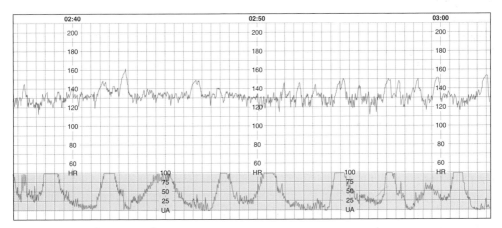

**Figure 64.1** Cardiotocograph.

### Questions
- What is the diagnosis?
- How should this woman be managed?

## ANSWER 64

The diagnosis is of placental abruption in view of the bleeding, uterine tenderness and irritability. CTG is reassuring at present with baseline 130 beats/min, normal variability, several accelerations and no decelerations. Regular uterine activity is demonstrated on the tocograph.

---

**!** **Common causes of antepartum haemorrhage (APH) at term**

- *Maternal blood:*
  - blood-stained show
  - bleeding placenta praevia
  - placental abruption
  - cervical ectropion
  - infection (e.g. candida)
- *Fetal blood:*
  - vasa praevia

---

A 'show' can be ruled out, as the blood is fresh rather than mucus-like and dark. Placenta praevia would have been detected at the anomaly scan, and bleeding placenta praevia is typically painless. She has no features suggesting infection, and vasa praevia bleeding would normally occur with rupture of membranes. Placental abruption is supported by the history of fresh bleeding and uterine irritability and the associated high blood pressure and proteinuria (pre-eclampsia is a cause of abruption).

Placental abruption may be major with catastrophic haemorrhage or, as in this case, be less dramatic. However, caution should be maintained for two reasons: first, a small bleed may herald a larger bleed. Second, although some bleeding is revealed, there may be a more significant concealed bleed. Pregnant women may not show any signs of hypovolaemic shock until a large amount of blood has been lost.

### Management

Women with APH should always be admitted for observation. Initial management for this woman includes intravenous access, group and save, full blood count and clotting profile. Urea, electrolytes and urate should be sent, looking for abnormalities associated with pre-eclampsia; 24-h urine collection for proteinuria is not indicated in this case as induction of labour is already indicated on clinical grounds. Blood pressure should be repeated at regular intervals and antihypertensives commenced if indicated.

Induction of labour may increase the chance of operative intervention, but the risk of expectant management is that sudden and catastrophic further haemorrhage may occur. As the woman is over 37 weeks, there is little risk to the fetus of prematurity from induction.

---

 **KEY POINTS**

- Placental abruption is a clinical diagnosis based on symptoms and examination.
- Blood loss caused by placental abruption may be concealed or revealed.
- A woman may not show signs of hypovolaemia until she had lost a large proportion of her blood volume.

---

# CASE 65: BREECH PRESENTATION

## History

You are asked to see a woman in the antenatal clinic. She is 37 years old and pregnant with her third child. Her previous children were both born by vaginal delivery after induction of labour for post dates.

First-trimester ultrasound confirmed her menstrual dates and she is now 37 weeks. At her last appointment at 36 weeks' gestation, the midwife suspected that the baby was in a breech presentation. An appointment has been made for an ultrasound assessment and to discuss the situation.

## Examination

Blood pressure is 140/85 mmHg and abdominal examination suggests a breech presentation with the sacrum not engaged.

---

### 🔍 INVESTIGATIONS

Urinalysis: negative

*Ultrasound report*:

Indication for scan: suspected breech presentation

Gestational age: 37 weeks 3 days

Frank breech presentation (hips flexed, knees straight)

Estimated fetal weight 3.2 kg

Placenta: high anterior

Liquor volume: normal (amniotic fluid index 18 cm).

---

## Questions
- What are the options available to the woman?
- What management would you recommend in this case?

# ANSWER 65

At 30 weeks the incidence of breech presentation is around 14 per cent, but is only 2–4 per cent by term.

| ! | Causes and associations for breech presentation |
|---|---|

- Grand multiparity (lax uterus)
- Uterine abnormality (bicornuate, septate, fibroids)
- Placenta praevia
- Polyhydramnios
- Oligohydramnios
- Multiple pregnancy
- Congenital fetal abnormality
- Prematurity

The three options available are:

1 external cephalic version
2 elective Caesarean section
3 vaginal breech delivery.

All three options should be discussed with the woman and her partner with important counselling points.

- *Vaginal breech delivery*:
  - found to be less safe for singleton term fetuses than planned Caesarean section
  - carries a high chance of necessitating an emergency Caesarean section
  - needs involvement of an experienced obstetrician with continuous fetal heart monitoring and ideally an epidural
  - should only be allowed if the labour progresses spontaneously – augmentation of breech labour is generally not recommended
  - contraindicated with placenta praevia, large baby, footling breech or maternal condition such as pre-eclampsia
- *External cephalic version*:
  - involves using external manipulation of the fetus, encouraging the baby to turn to the cephalic presentation by way of pressure on the maternal abdomen
  - is often performed after giving a uterine relaxant such as salbutamol
  - carries a very small chance of abnormal fetal heart rate during or after the procedure which could necessitate an emergency Caesarean section
  - has approximately 50 per cent success rate overall
  - some fetuses revert to breech position even after successful external cephalic version
  - contraindicated with previous Caesarean section, other uterine surgery, pre-eclampsia, intrauterine growth retardation, oligohydramnios
  - can be painful
- *Elective Caesarean section*:
  - is safer than vaginal breech delivery
  - is suitable where contraindications exist to external cephalic version
  - can be planned for in advance, which women may find more convenient
  - does not necessarily mean a woman would need a Caesarean section for any future pregnancy.

In this case the woman should be recommended external cephalic version as soon as possible, with options for an elective Caesarean section or possible trial of breech delivery if this is unsuccessful.

Postnatal paediatric review should focus on the baby's hips, with a neonatal ultrasound arranged within 6 weeks to rule out congenital hip dislocation (10–15 times more common in breech presentation).

 **KEY POINTS**

- Breech presentation is associated with increased perinatal morbidity and mortality.
- If a woman has a frank breech at 37 weeks she should normally be offered external cephalic version, and if unsuccessful an elective Caesarean section or possibly a vaginal breech delivery.

# CASE 66: ANTENATAL SCREENING

## History

A 31-year-old pregnant Russian woman came to the UK 6 weeks ago with her English husband. As a result she booked late with the midwife at 31 weeks' gestation. This is her first ongoing pregnancy, having had two uncomplicated surgical terminations approximately 10 years ago. She reports a history of genital herpes diagnosed by her general practitioner several weeks ago. There is no relevant previous general medical history or family history.

She had an apparently normal first-trimester scan in Russia before arriving in the UK and has had a normal anomaly scan in this hospital at 30 weeks' gestation.

## Examination

Blood pressure is normal and symphysiofundal height is consistent with menstrual dates.

---

**🔍 INVESTIGATIONS**

| | | *Normal range for pregnancy* |
|---|---|---|
| Haemoglobin | 11.7 g/dL | 11–14 g/dL |
| Mean cell volume | 87 fL | 74.4–95.6 fL |
| White cell count | $10.4 \times 10^9$/L | $6$–$16 \times 10^9$/L |
| Platelets | $389 \times 10^9$/L | $150$–$400 \times 10^9$/L |

Blood group: AB positive

Hepatitis B antigen: negative

Rubella antibody: immune

HIV1/2: negative

*T. pallidum* enzyme immunoassay (EIA): positive.

---

## Questions
- What is the diagnosis?
- How should the woman be further investigated and treated?

## ANSWER 66

Screening for syphilis is recommended for all pregnant women and *T. pallidum* EIA is a specific test for syphilis infection. The prevalence of infection is up to 0.3/1000 pregnant women in the UK. EIA tests that detect immunoglobulin G (IgG) or IgG and IgM, *T. pallidum* haemagglutination test and the fluorescent treponemal antibody-absorbed test (FTA-abs) are used generally for screening in pregnancy, as they are 98 per cent sensitive and over 99 per cent specific.

In cases with a positive screening test a second treponemal-specific confirmatory test should be sent to confirm the diagnosis. Caution is needed as treponemal-specific tests cannot differentiate syphilis from other treponemal disease (yaws, pinta and bejel).

The diagnosis in this woman is syphilis infection. She should be referred to a genito-urinary medicine clinic for urgent assessment and treatment. She may have a genital ulcer (possibly misdiagnosed as herpes simplex by her doctor) or features of secondary syphilis, but many women diagnosed are asymptomatic (latent syphilis).

### Management

Treatment is with intramuscular penicillin daily for 10 days (doxycycline or erythromycin if penicillin allergic). Follow-up with a quantitative test (such as venereal disease research laboratory [VDRL] should be used to confirm effective treatment and to monitor for reinfection. The woman's partner should be referred to the genitourinary medicine clinic for testing (45–60 per cent of partners will be infected).

The paediatricians should be informed at delivery to assess for signs of early congenital syphilis (usually developing in the first few weeks of life) and to arrange serological testing.

Untreated, 70–100 per cent of babies of mothers with syphilis infection will develop congenital syphilis, with a 30 per cent stillbirth rate.

---

**!  Features of congenital syphilis**

- Early congenital syphilis due to transplacental transfer of organisms (<2 years):
  - condylomata lata rash
  - snuffles
  - lymphadenopathy
  - hepatosplenomegaly
  - ocular, renal and haematological involvement
- Late congenital syphilis due to early structural damage (>2 years)
  - interstitial keratitis
  - Hutchinson's incisors
  - Clutton's joints
  - saddle nose deformity
  - frontal bossing
  - deafness.

---

 **KEY POINTS**

- *T. pallidum* EIA is an enzyme immunoassay for syphilis.
- If untreated, pregnant women with syphilis will have a 30 per cent chance of a stillbirth and 70–100 per cent chance that the baby will have been infected with syphilis.

# CASE 67: PAIN IN PREGNANCY

## History

A 40-year-old woman presents with a fever and abdominal pain. She is 18 weeks pregnant in her third pregnancy. The pregnancy has been unremarkable so far and she has no significant gynaecological or medical history.

She has felt unwell for 10 days but has become worse in the last 48 h. She is nauseated and has vomited several times. She is intermittently hot and cold. Her abdominal pain is generalized and constant with some right-sided loin pain.

She denies any dysuria and says that she has frequency which has been present throughout the pregnancy. She has had no recent change in bowel habit. There has been no vaginal bleeding and she has a mild thin vaginal discharge.

## Examination

She appears flushed and unwell. Her temperature is 38.2°C, blood pressure 115/68 mmHg and pulse 112/min. Cardiac and chest examination is normal. The fundal height is approximately 2 cm below the umbilicus, and the uterus is soft and non-tender. The rest of the abdomen is tender on deep palpation, maximally in the right lower quadrant. There is right renal angle tenderness. The fetal heart is heard at 160/min with hand-held Doppler.

| INVESTIGATIONS | | |
|---|---|---|
| | | Normal range for pregnancy |
| Haemoglobin | 11.1 g/dL | 11–14 g/dL |
| White cell count | 18.9 × 10⁹/L | 6–16 × 10⁹/L |
| Neutrophils | 16.2 × 10⁹/L | 2–7.5 × 10⁹/L |
| Platelets | 346 × 10⁹/L | 150–400 × 10⁹/L |
| Sodium | 139 mmol/L | 130–140 mmol/L |
| Potassium | 4.2 mmol/L | 3.3–4.1 mmol/L |
| Urea | 8.1 mmol/L | 2.4–4.3 mmol/L |
| Creatinine | 68 μmol/L | 34–82 μmol/L |
| C-reactive protein | 127 mg/L | <5 mg/L |

Urinalysis: + protein; + blood; ++ leucocytes; + nitrites.

## Questions

• What is the diagnosis?
• How would you investigate and manage this woman?

# ANSWER 67

The diagnosis is of pyelonephritis, which occurs in 1–2 per cent of pregnancies. Women can be very unwell with non-specific symptoms. In this case specific factors are evident (loin pain and positive urinalysis).

Urinary tract infections (UTIs) are common in pregnancy due to progesterone causing stasis of urine and pressure of the gravid uterus causing ureteric obstruction.

## Further investigation

The diagnosis should be confirmed with urine microscopy, culture and sensitivity, and blood cultures should be sent prior to commencing antibiotics. Renal tract ultrasound scan is necessary to rule out any congenital abnormality (such as duplex ureters) that may predispose to renal tract infection, and to rule out an infected obstructed kidney which could need urgent drainage by nephrostomy. Renal tract ultrasound, however, can be difficult to interpret in pregnancy as physiological dilatation of the ureters occurs from pressure from the uterus.

## Management

Intravenous antibiotics should be started, usually cephalosporins, until culture and sensitivities are available, with regular paracetamol to control the temperature and pain. It may take several days for the temperature to settle and for the woman's pain and symptoms to resolve, but improvement should be monitored with daily white blood count, C-reactive protein and urea and electrolytes. Intravenous rehydration is needed as the woman is vomiting and pyrexial with raised urea, suggesting dehydration.

After completion of treatment (total 2 weeks) a repeat urine culture is needed to confirm cure. Some women with recurrent infection need a daily prophylactic antibiotic regime.

## Effect on the pregnancy

Maternal sepsis is a risk for miscarriage and preterm labour, so treatment should not be delayed. In addition, recurrent UTI, even asymptomatic bacteriuria, is associated with intrauterine growth retardation and preterm labour.

---

 **KEY POINTS**

- Urinary tract infections are common in pregnancy.
- Pyelonephritis must be treated aggressively with intravenous antibiotics to avoid miscarriage or preterm delivery.

---

## CASE 68: POSTPARTUM CHEST PAIN

### History

A 32-year-old Sri Lankan woman presents complaining of chest pain, neck tightness and shortness of breath 3 weeks after delivery. The symptoms have come on gradually over the last 2 days and are now severe. She feels as if she cannot breathe and thinks she is going to die.

The pain is heavy and stabbing and is constant though worse when she lies down and tries to sleep. The pain is not pleuritic and she says it radiates up into her neck. She does not have a cough or haemoptysis.

The neck tightness is all over the neck but especially anteriorly, and is related to the difficulty breathing. There is no photophobia or fever.

The breathing difficulty occurs predominantly when she is trying to sleep or is sleeping – it has woken her several times during the night. She is now terrified of going to sleep and is actively stopping herself from doing so as she is certain that she will die if she does.

Prior to this she has always been fit and well with no previous medical history reported.

The pregnancy was uneventful and she was admitted in spontaneous labour at 40 weeks. Cervical dilatation was slow and contractions were therefore augmented with syntocinon. Once fully dilated she had pushed for 90 min and subsequently underwent ventouse delivery of a healthy female infant.

She had some difficulty establishing breast-feeding and bonding with the baby and was finally discharged home on day four following delivery. Since going home she has stopped breast-feeding but is finding it difficult to sleep even when the baby is sleeping.

She has lived in the UK for 18 months but her husband has been here for 6 years. Currently her mother is also staying with them to help with the baby. Both the woman and her mother speak very little English and the husband is interpreting.

### Examination

She is thin and quiet, with little eye contact. When talking about the baby she is non-responsive and she does not look at or touch the baby during the consultation. Her blood pressure is 108/62 mmHg and heart rate 90/min. She is apyrexial. There are no signs of anaemia, cyanosis or oedema. Chest and cardiac examination are normal and the uterus is just palpable in the lower abdomen.

| INVESTIGATIONS | | |
|---|---|---|
| | | *Normal range for pregnancy* |
| Haemoglobin | 10.8 g/dL | 11–14 g/dL |
| Mean cell volume | 78 fL | 74.4–95.6 fL |
| White cell count | $5.3 \times 10^9$/L | $6–16 \times 10^9$/L |
| Platelets | $237 \times 10^9$/L | $150–400 \times 10^9$/L |

Electrocardiogram (ECG): sinus rhythm, no abnormalities

Chest X-ray: normal heart and lung fields

Oxygen saturation: 100 per cent on air

*Arterial blood gas:*

| | | |
|---|---|---|
| $pO_2$ | 16 kPa | 12–14 kPa |
| $pCO_2$ | 3.8 kPa | 5–6 kPa |

### Questions

- What is the likely diagnosis?
- What further questions would you wish to ask and what are the principles of management?

# ANSWER 68

The symptoms initially sound possibly cardiac or respiratory in origin. However, the story does not fit with any specific disease and the examination and investigations are all normal. The absolute fear of sleeping is an important piece of information as is the reported affect.

This woman is suffering from postnatal psychosis. This occurs in 1 in 500 women with onset in the first 6 weeks post delivery. The commonest symptoms are delusions (e.g. the thought that she is going to die) and hallucinations.

The condition should be distinguished from the two other main psychological/psychiatric postnatal conditions.

- *Post-partum blues*:
  - tearfulness
  - fatigue
  - anxiety over their own or the baby's health
  - feelings of inability to cope

This is very common (probably affecting approximately half of mothers) usually after the third postnatal day, and resolves spontaneously over a few days.

- *Post-partum depression*:
  - low mood
  - crying
  - anxiety over the baby's health
  - feelings of guilt towards the baby
  - panic attacks
  - excessive tiredness
  - poor appetite

This occurs in 10 per cent of women, any time up to 6 months following delivery. It should be treated seriously with suicide risk assessment and antidepressant medication as well as social and practical support.

## Further questioning

A trained interpreter should be sought rather than the husband who is involved in this case and may find it difficult to translate or address sensitive issues.

The woman should be asked for any previous personal or family history of mental illness or psychiatric treatment. She should then be asked more probing questions. How is her mood and appetite? Does she feel depressed? Does she have fears of harming herself?

Her relationship and attitudes to the baby are important – how does she feel about the baby? Is she finding the baby easy? Does she feel that the baby is healthy? Does she have any negative thoughts toward the baby such that it is bad or evil? Does she feel she might harm the baby?

Suicide is now the commonest cause of indirect maternal death, and non-English-speaking immigrants are particularly at risk as well as those aged over 30 years, with previous psychotic history, poor social support or traumatic delivery. This woman has three such risk factors.

The diagnosis should always be considered when symptoms do not appear to be backed up by the examination or investigations. Sometimes delusional symptoms or hallucinations are not elicited because the doctor fails to take a thorough history.

## Management

Disease progression can be acute and this woman needs immediate referral to a mother and baby psychiatric unit for assessment and treatment. Depending on her feelings of harm towards herself or others, this may need to be under the Mental Health Act. Antidepressants, antipsychotics and possibly sedation may be needed. The baby may be at risk from neglect or harm secondary to the psychosis, so close supervision and support is essential. Recovery is expected within 2 months but repeat pregnancy and non-pregnancy-related episodes are common.

 **KEY POINTS**

- Postpartum psychosis is generally diagnosed in the community after discharge from hospital after delivery.
- Women with postpartum psychosis must be admitted to a mother and baby psychiatric unit, if need be under the Mental Health Act.

# CASE 69: ANTI-D

### History

A couple attends the obstetric clinic at 20 weeks' gestation. This is the woman's fourth pregnancy and second child. She is 27 years old. She had a spontaneous vaginal delivery 4 years ago and this was followed by two miscarriages, the first at 8 weeks and the second at 14 weeks, for which no cause was identified.

In this pregnancy she has been generally well except for severe hyperemesis which has now resolved. Her 11–14-week scan confirmed her menstrual dates and she was given a risk of Down's syndrome from her nuchal test of 1 in 2543. Her anomaly scan has just been performed and shows no fetal abnormalities, and normal fetal growth and liquor volume.

She is known to be Rhesus negative and her booking and subsequent haematological blood tests are as shown.

### INVESTIGATIONS

| | | Normal range for pregnancy |
|---|---|---|
| *Booking* | | |
| Haemoglobin | 13.1 g/dL | 11–14 g/dL |
| White cell count | $7.0 \times 10^9$/L | $6–16 \times 10^9$/L |
| Platelets | $226 \times 10^9$/L | $150–400 \times 10^9$/L |

Blood group: O negative

Anti-D antibodies: present (titre 4 IU/mL)

*16 weeks*

Anti-D antibodies: present (titre 4 IU/mL)

*20 weeks*

Anti-D antibodies: present (titre 9 IU/mL).

### Questions
- What is the diagnosis?
- What are the potential consequences of this problem?
- How would you further manage the pregnancy?

# ANSWER 69

The diagnosis is Rhesus sensitization as the serum anti-D titre is increasing, suggesting that sometime exposure to Rhesus positive cells has sensitized her, causing her to produce an immune response (anti-D). This may have occurred if she was not given anti-D at the time of a previous pregnancy.

## Consequences

Immunoglobulin G (IgG) anti-D antibodies cross the placenta and attack fetal Rhesus-positive red cells. This causes fetal haemolysis (haemolytic disease of the newborn or the fetus) manifesting as fetal anaemia, with subsequent fetal hydrops (excessive accumulation of extravascular fluid e.g. peritoneal, pleural, pericardial). Intrauterine death may occur if the anaemia is not treated. In milder cases, the baby may be severely jaundiced at delivery, which may result in neurological impairment. For the mother there is a potential difficulty crossmatching blood should she have a haemorrhagic complication and need transfusion, due to the presence of the antibodies.

## Management

The maternal antibody level should be monitored two weekly. If the titre exceeds 15 IU/mL, fetal ultrasound should be performed to assess for growth retardation, signs of hydrops and liquor volume. Cordocentesis (sampling fetal blood by ultrasound-guided aspiration from the umbilical cord) is needed to determine haemoglobin and to facilitate fetal blood transfusion. If the antibody titre does not increase further then ultrasound observation is likely to be sufficient.

In this case, the antibody titre was 15 IU/mL 2 weeks later and the fetus required three in utero transfusions during the pregnancy, with delivery by Caesarean section at 36 weeks.

Fifteen per cent of women are Rhesus negative, but due to anti-D prophylaxis, the incidence of Rhesus disease is now very low.

---

 **Potential sensitizing events for rhesus disease**

- Miscarriage, ectopic pregnancy, termination
- Abdominal trauma, invasive tests (e.g. amniocentesis) or external cephalic version
- Placental abruption
- Delivery
- Rhesus-positive blood transfusion to a Rhesus-negative woman

Anti-D previously was given after any potentially sensitizing event, but is now routinely given at 28 and 34 weeks' gestation. Anti-D should not be given to a woman who has already developed anti-D antibodies.

---

### KEY POINTS

- Rhesus disease is now rare due to anti-D prophylaxis; however, we must be vigilant to events that may sensitize a woman.

# CASE 70: HIV IN PREGNANCY

## History

A 36-year-old Nigerian woman who has lived in the UK for 8 years attends the antenatal clinic. She had a daughter by spontaneous vaginal delivery at term 12 years ago and a termination of pregnancy 9 years ago. She and her partner have now been trying to conceive for 4 years.

Her last menstrual period was 11 weeks ago. There is no significant gynaecological history and last smear test was normal 2 years ago.

The woman saw the midwife for a routine antenatal booking appointment a week ago and no relevant past medical history was reported. All routine booking blood tests were accepted.

---

### INVESTIGATIONS

|  |  | Normal range for pregnancy |
|---|---|---|
| Haemoglobin | 11.9 g/dL | 11–14 g/dL |
| Mean cell volume | 77 fL | 74.4–95.6 fL |
| White count | $4.1 \times 10^9$/L | $6–16 \times 10^9$/L |
| Platelets | $129 \times 10^9$/L | $150–400 \times 10^9$/L |

Blood group: AB positive

Hepatitis B surface antigen: negative

Syphilis: negative

HIV1/2: positive

Rubella: immune

CD4: 175/mm$^3$

Viral load: 10 000 copies/mL

---

## Questions

- What is the diagnosis?
- What is the next stage in management?
- What are the important points in the management of the pregnancy in view of the diagnosis?

# ANSWER 70

The diagnosis is human immunodeficiency virus (HIV) infection. HIV screening in pregnancy is recommended for all women in the UK and the latest reported incidence was approximately 0.5 per cent in inner London and less than 0.1 per cent for the rest of the UK. It is particularly prevalent in women from Africa (1.91 per cent compared with <0.5 per cent from all other areas). The vast majority of paediatric HIV cases in the UK result from mother-to-child transmission.

The low CD4 count suggests that this woman needs to commence treatment, but there are no AIDS-defining illnesses in the history.

## Immediate management

The woman needs to be informed of the diagnosis and a second different diagnostic test performed to confirm the diagnosis. Most women choose to continue with their pregnancies, but she may still wish to consider the option of termination, as she is only 11 weeks' gestation. She needs urgent referral to the genitourinary medicine specialist for further examination and investigation for any HIV complications. She will need to start *Pneumocystis carinii* prophylaxis in view of the low CD4 count, and she will also need antiretroviral treatment in view of the significant viral load.

Psychological counselling in relation to the diagnosis, the implications for her, her partner and her offspring (the fetus and her 12-year-old daughter) is very important.

## Management of the pregnancy

Pregnancy does not adversely affect the HIV disease process. The important consideration is therefore the prevention of transmission from mother to child. Untreated, approximately 25 per cent of infants of mothers with HIV will become infected. With appropriate measures, this is reduced to less than 5 per cent:

- elective Caesarean section
- avoidance of breast-feeding
- intravenous zidovudine to the mother prior to delivery (ideally for 4 h)
- oral zidovudine to the neonate for 6 weeks postnatally.

More recently, vaginal delivery has been shown to have no effect on infant infection if the viral load is undetectable at the time of delivery.

Confidentiality is of paramount importance for women diagnosed antenatally with HIV, and coding systems in the hand-held obstetric notes can be helpful in alerting other medical staff to the diagnosis.

---

 **KEY POINTS**

- The incidence of HIV in pregnancy is increasing.
- To decrease vertical transmission the mother should have an elective Caesarean section, avoid breast-feeding, have intravenous zidovudine prior to delivery and the neonate should be given zidovudine for 6 weeks.

---

# CASE 71: ITCHING IN PREGNANCY

## History

A 36-year-old woman is complaining of itching. She is currently 34 weeks' gestation in her first ongoing pregnancy, having had two previous early miscarriages. The itching started 2 weeks ago and she had been using emollient cream to try and relieve it. Initially it was mainly over her soles and palms, although it is now more generalized. She is not aware of having changed her washing powder or soap recently and no one else in her family has been affected.

She has not experienced any abdominal pain although she does have Braxton Hicks contractions. There is no vaginal discharge or bleeding. She has noticed the baby move more than 10 times in the last 12 h.

## Examination

She looks well. Her blood pressure is 118/76 mmHg and pulse 82/min.

No rash is visible on the face, trunk, limbs, hands or feet except for a few excoriation marks.

The symphysiofundal height is 34.5 cm and the uterus is soft and non-tender. The fetus is cephalic with 4/5 palpable abdominally.

| INVESTIGATIONS | | |
|---|---|---|
| | | Normal for pregnancy |
| Haemoglobin | 10.3 g/dL | 11–14 g/dL |
| Mean cell volume | 80 fL | 74.4–95.6 fL |
| Platelets | 198 × 10⁹/L | 150–400 × 10⁹/L |
| Sodium | 132 mmol/L | 130–140 mmol/L |
| Potassium | 3.3 mmol/L | 3.3–4.1 mmol/L |
| Urea | 2.9 mmol/L | 2.4–4.3 mmol/L |
| Creatinine | 68 µmol/L | 34–82 µmol/L |
| Alanine transaminase | 31 IU/L | 6–32 IU/L |
| Alkaline phosphatase | 120 IU/L | 30–300 IU/L |
| Gamma glutamyl transaminase | 12 IU/L | 5–43 IU/L |
| Bilirubin | 8 µmol/L | 3–14 µmol/L |
| Bile acid | 24 µmol/L | 0–14 µmol/L |

Urinalysis: nil abnormal detected.

## Questions

- What is the diagnosis?
- How would you further investigate and manage this woman?
- How will this diagnosis affect the pregnancy?

# ANSWER 71

The woman is suffering from obstetric cholestasis (OC). This is a pregnancy-specific condition in which there is intrahepatic reduction of bile excretion from the liver, causing a build-up of serum bile acids. It usually develops in the third trimester. The effect on the mother is of itching, which may be very distressing. In more severe cases the liver function or coagulation become deranged and if they do then other diagnoses such as HELLP syndrome (haemolysis, elevated liver enzymes and low platelets – a severe form of pre-eclampsia) or hepatitis should be considered. An ultrasound should be performed to exclude other causes of obstruction such as gallstones.

There is no long-term harm to the mother. The effect on the baby however is potentially much more serious with an association between OC and stillbirth.

## Investigations
Liver ultrasound should be performed to exclude other causes of hepatic obstruction. Fetal ultrasound may be performed for maternal reassurance.

## Management
Symptomatic relief is obtained from chlorpheniramine (antihistamine). Ursodeoxycholic acid can be given to relieve itching in more severe cases, as it reduces serum bile acids.

Vitamin K (needed for clotting factors) should be given orally to the mother to reduce the risk of fetal or maternal haemorrhage caused by impaired absorption.

## Postnatal advice
Maternal liver function returns to normal after delivery, but the mother should be warned that recurrence may occur in a subsequent pregnancy (50 per cent) or with use of the combined oral contraceptive pill.

---

 **KEY POINTS**

- Itching in pregnancy may be due to obstetric cholestasis.
- In severe cases maternal liver and coagulation function can become deranged, but usually the major risk is to the fetus.
- There is a high risk (50 per cent) of recurrence in future pregnancies.

---

# CASE 72: TIREDNESS IN PREGNANCY

## History

A 27-year-old woman attends the antenatal clinic at 19 weeks' gestation in her first ongoing pregnancy, having had a termination aged 22 years. She is now happy to be pregnant.

She booked with the midwife at 8 weeks and has had normal booking bloods, blood pressure and ultrasound scan.

She experienced nausea and vomiting until 14 weeks' gestation. This has now settled but she remains very tired and feels that she is gaining excessive weight in the pregnancy. She also feels cold for much of the time, which surprises her as she understood that pregnant women tend to feel hot.

## Examination

The woman appears lethargic and of low mood. Her blood pressure is 115/68 mmHg and heart rate 58/min. Abdominal examination is unremarkable, with the fundus palpable at the umbilicus.

| INVESTIGATIONS | | |
|---|---|---|
| | | Normal range for pregnancy |
| Haemoglobin | 10.2 g/dL | 11–14 g/dL |
| Mean cell volume | 78 fL | 74.4–95.6 fL |
| White cell count | $7.9 \times 10^9$/L | $6–16 \times 10^9$/L |
| Platelets | $272 \times 10^9$/L | $150–400 \times 10^9$/L |
| Thyroid-stimulating hormone (TSH) antibody | 15 mu/L | 0.5–7 mu/L |
| Free thyroxine ($T_4$) | 6 pmol/L | 11–23 pmol/L |

## Questions

- What is the diagnosis and what features will you look for on examination?
- What are the implications for the mother and baby in pregnancy?
- How should the condition be managed?

# ANSWER 72

The full blood count shows mild anaemia, with relatively low mean cell volume. This is not significant enough to account for the symptoms described.

The thyroid function tests confirm the clinical diagnosis of hypothyroidism. There is no history of radioactive iodine or surgical treatment, and Hashimoto's thyroiditis is unlikely as there has been no history of a hyperthyroid episode. This case therefore probably represents idiopathic myxoedema.

The symptoms of tiredness, cold intolerance and weight gain may all relate to the hypo-thyroidism. In addition she may report dry skin, coarse hair, depression or constipation.

Examination may reveal relative bradycardia, blunted deep tendon reflexes or goitre.

## Implications for the pregnancy and management
Hypothyroidism occurs in approximately 1 in 100 pregnancies, but this case is unusual to be diagnosed in pregnancy.

Myxoedematous coma is a very rare consequence of hypothyroidism, associated with a high mortality rate. It is a medical emergency managed by supportive care and thyroxine supplementation. In the absence of a coma, thyroxine replacement is still needed and should be titrated to the TSH and $T_4$ results.

In pregnancy, the thyroxine requirement may increase, and the TSH and $T_4$ should be checked every trimester once a maintenance regime has been established. The aim should be to keep the TSH less than 5 mu/L.

(Although the thyroid-binding globulin increases in pregnancy, there is a compensatory rise in tri-iodothyronine ($T_3$) and $T_4$ production such that the levels of free $T_3$ and free $T_4$ remain similar to non-pregnant values.)

## The fetus
Untreated hypothyroidism is associated with an increased risk of infertility, miscarriage, stillbirth and pre-eclampsia. The fetal and neonatal outcome is generally good in women diagnosed and treated appropriately. Anti-TSH antibodies may very rarely cross the pla-centa and cause neonatal hypothyroidism, and this should be suspected if there are signs of neonatal goitre.

---

 **KEY POINTS**

- Untreated hypothyroidism is associated with infertility, miscarriage, low birth weight, fetal loss, pre-eclampsia and anaemia.
- Women established on thyroxine should have thyroid function monitored once in each trimester of pregnancy.

## CASE 73: DIABETES IN PREGNANCY

### History

A 20-year-old woman is pregnant for the first time. The pregnancy is unplanned and the partner has left but she is supported by her mother and has decided to continue.

She was diagnosed with type 1 diabetes aged 15 years. She has been taking long-acting and short-acting insulin under the care of her general practitioner (GP), but the referral letter suggests that she has not always been compliant.

She had a positive pregnancy test 2 weeks ago and her GP has referred her urgently to the antenatal clinic for review in view of the diabetes. By her dates she is now 7 weeks and 5 days' gestation. She has no other significant gynaecological or medical history.

### Examination

The woman has a body mass index of $29 \, \text{kg/m}^2$. Blood pressure is 131/68 mmHg and pulse is 81/min.

| INVESTIGATIONS | | |
|---|---|---|
| | | *Normal* |
| Haemoglobin (Hb)A$_{1c}$ | 7.8% | <7.0% |
| Urinalysis: ++ glucose. | | |

### Questions
- What further investigations need to be arranged?
- Outline the principles of management of the pregnancy.

# ANSWER 73

The investigations can be divided into those for maternal and for fetal wellbeing:

- *maternal wellbeing*:
  - baseline urea and electrolytes
  - pre- and post-prandial capillary blood glucose measurements
- *fetal wellbeing*:
  - viability scan (increased risk of miscarriage in diabetic women)
  - fetal echocardiography (increased risk of all fetal abnormalities in diabetic offspring)
  - detailed anomaly ultrasound examination at 20 weeks.

Diabetic (type 1) pregnancies may be affected by an increase in a range of complications as well as fetal abnormalities. However optimal control of blood sugar is thought to reduce the complication risk to near that of a non-diabetic pregnancy, so a large proportion of management is aimed at maintaining very tight blood glucose control. In this particular case, the history, $HbA_{1c}$ and presence of glycosuria suggest that the woman has generally poor control, providing a particular challenge to management of this pregnancy.

---

**!** | **Management principles in maternal insulin-dependent diabetes**

- *Antenatal*:
  - immediate change to an increased insulin-dosing regime using more frequent doses to adapt to the increasing demand in pregnancy
  - multidisciplinary care with endocrinologist/diabetologist, dietitian, specialist diabetic nurse, obstetrician and midwife with special interest in diabetic pregnancies
  - full hospital care with regular review, usually every 2 weeks, or more frequently if control remains poor
  - increase in insulin requirements expected throughout the pregnancy
  - regular ultrasound assessment from 28 weeks for fetal growth and liquor volume, in view of the risk of macrosomia and polyhydramnios, secondary to fetal hyperinsulinaemia
  - consideration of induction of labour at 38 weeks to reduce the risk of sudden stillbirth
- *In labour*:
  - sliding-scale insulin regime in labour (or during Caesarean section)
  - aim for vaginal delivery unless contraindicated by obstetric factors
- *Postnatal*:
  - early blood glucose checks and feeding of the baby in view of its hyperinsulinaemic state
  - reduction of maternal insulin regime to the pre-pregnancy regime immediately after delivery

---

**KEY POINTS**

- Type 1 diabetes pregnancies are high risk for mother and fetus and need specialist diabetes and obstetric input. Very close blood glucose control should reduce the complication rate to near that of a non-diabetic mother.
- Fetal complications include miscarriage, congenital abnormality, macrosomia, stillbirth and shoulder dystocia.

# PERIPARTUM CARE AND OBSTETRIC EMERGENCIES

## CASE 74: ABSENT FETAL MOVEMENTS

### History

A 34-year-old woman at 32 weeks and 4 days' gestation in her first pregnancy complains of reduced fetal movements. She normally feels the baby move more than 10 times each day but yesterday there were only two movements and today there have been none. She has no significant medical, obstetric or gynaecological history. In this pregnancy she booked at 10 weeks' gestation and all her booking blood tests were normal except that she was discovered not to be immune to rubella and postnatal vaccination was planned. Her 11–14-week scan, nuchal translucency test and anomaly scan were all normal.

### Examination

The blood pressure is 137/73 mmHg and pulse 93/min. She is apyrexial. The symphysio-fundal height of the uterus is 31 cm and the fetus is breech on examination. The fetal heart is auscultated with hand-held Doppler and no heartbeat is heard. An ultrasound scan is therefore arranged immediately, which confirms the diagnosis of intrauterine fetal death.

### Questions

- How should this case be managed?
- Are there any factors in the history or examination to indicate the cause of fetal death and what investigations should be performed to establish a possible cause?

# ANSWER 74

### Immediate management

The baby needs delivery to avoid the possibility of sepsis or disseminated intravascular coagulopathy developing. This is normally achieved by induction of labour with mifepristone (an antiprogestogen) followed 48 h later by misoprostol (a prostaglandin analogue) to induce contractions. The woman can go home temporarily after the mifepristone to avoid the added stress from being on an antenatal or postnatal ward.

In labour, adequate analgesia is essential and patient-controlled analgesia (PCA) is useful.

Rarely there are contraindications to vaginal delivery, such as previous Caesarean sections, in which case operative delivery may be necessary.

The couple should be seen as soon as possible by a bereavement midwife to discuss the loss, funeral or cremation plans.

### Cause of intrauterine death

In this history the only potentially significant factor is the lack of rubella immunity. This is unlikely to be significant, but rubella immunoglobulin (IgG) should be checked to exclude recent infection.

The examination is normal except for the tachycardia, which may relate to anxiety and should be rechecked.

---

**！ Possible causes of intrauterine death**

- *Maternal*:
  - diabetes
  - infection (e.g. parvovirus, listeria)
  - thrombophilia (e.g. antiphospholipid syndrome)
- *Fetal*:
  - chromosomal abnormality (e.g. trisomy)
  - other genetic abnormality (e.g. Gaucher's disease)
  - haemolytic disease
  - cord incident (eg 'knot' in cord)
- *Placental*:
  - placental abruption
  - uteroplacental insufficiency (e.g. secondary to pre-eclampsia)
  - postmaturity
- *Unexplained*

---

### Investigations

- *Maternal*:
  - full blood count and coagulation screen (to exclude disseminated intravascular coagulopathy/thrombocytopenia secondary to fetal death)
  - random blood glucose and haemoglobin (Hb)$A_{1c}$
  - Kleihauer test (for fetal cells in the maternal circulation, implying significant fetomaternal haemorrhage)
  - anticardiolipin and lupus anticoagulant (for antiphospholipid syndrome)

- *Fetal*:
  - swabs for microscopy, culture and sensitivity from the fetus and placenta
  - skin biopsy for karyotype
  - post mortem (if agreed by parents)

| KEY POINTS |
| --- |
| • Intrauterine death is commonly unexpected and unexplained. <br> • Induction of labour should be arranged as soon as possible as there is a risk of the development of sepsis or disseminated intravascular coagulopathy. |

# CASE 75: LABOUR

## History
You are on the labour ward and called to see a 33-year-old woman in labour as the midwife is concerned about the cardiotocograph (CTG).

She is 41 + 2 weeks' gestation and this is her first baby. The pregnancy was uncomplicated until 2 days ago when she developed mild hypertension, without proteinuria. In view of the gestational age a decision was made for induction of labour yesterday. She had 2 mg prostaglandin gel administered into the vagina at 18.00 last night and again at 06.00 this morning. Spontaneous rupture of membranes occurred at 10.00 today after which contractions commenced.

## Examination
Blood pressure is 135/68 mmHg, heart rate 90/min and temperature is 37.1°C.

On abdominal palpation the fetus is cephalic, 1/5 palpable, and strong contractions are felt. Vaginally the cervix is fully effaced and 6 cm dilated. The fetus is cephalic at ischial spines with mild caput but no moulding. Grade 1 meconium is noted.

---

### 🔍 INVESTIGATIONS

The CTG is shown in Fig. 75.1.

A decision is made for fetal blood sampling and the result is as follows:
pH: 7.10

Base excess: −7.9 mmol/L

---

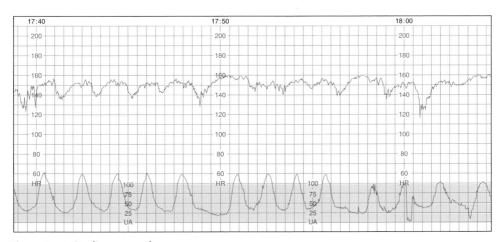

**Figure 75.1** Cardiotocograph.

## Questions
- How would you interpret the CTG and fetal blood sample result?
- How would you manage the patient?

# ANSWER 75

The CTG shows a baseline of 155 beats/min with reduced variability (5–10 beats/min) and late decelerations. No accelerations are seen. The CTG is therefore classified as abnormal. Contractions are 5 in 10.

| ❗ Definition of a late deceleration |
| --- |
| A reduction in fetal heart rate from baseline of at least 15 beats for at least 15s |

The fetal pH should normally be between 7.25 and 7.35. This fetal blood sample suggests an acidotic baby (low pH and high negative base excess).

In cases of an abnormal CTG, the fetus may not be compromised, and it is therefore important to assess the fetal wellbeing with a fetal blood sample before progressing to operative intervention (unless fetal blood sampling is contraindicated or in cases of persistent fetal bradycardia). In this case the fetal blood sample confirmed that the fetus was significantly compromised.

The meconium-stained liquor may be a sign of fetal compromise, but at 41 weeks' gestation meconium may be an incidental finding and is therefore difficult to interpret.

## Management

If the cervix were fully dilated and the head below the ischial spines then instrumental delivery, by ventouse or forceps, would be appropriate. As this is not the case, then immediate delivery by Caesarean section is essential. The important points for an emergency Caesarean section are:

- the midwife in charge, theatre staff, obstetric consultant, specialist registrar, anaesthetist and paediatrician should be informed
- the reasons for the proposed procedure should be explained to the woman and informed consent obtained
- metoclopramide and ranitidine should be given in case of the need for general anaesthetic
- intravenous access is needed with full blood count and group and save sent
- a urethral catheter should be inserted
- the baby should be delivered within a maximum 30 min after the decision.

|  KEY POINTS |
| --- |
| • Late decelerations in labour are abnormal.<br>• A fetal blood sample should be taken to confirm fetal status before proceeding to an operative delivery. |

# CASE 76: PERIPARTUM COLLAPSE

## History

A woman aged 28 years is in labour when she suddenly collapses. This is her fourth pregnancy and she has had three previous spontaneous vaginal deliveries at term. This pregnancy has been uncomplicated and she has been admitted with contractions at 37 weeks and 6 days.

On arrival on the labour ward the fetus was palpated to be normal size, cephalic and 3/5 palpable abdominally. The cervix was 3 cm dilated and the membranes were intact. Blood pressure and urinalysis were normal. Initial auscultation of the fetus was reassuring and the heart rate has continued to be normal (around 140/min) on intermittent auscultation.

Five minutes ago spontaneous rupture of membranes occurred during a contraction, with a large gush of clear fluid from the vagina. The woman reported an urge to push at that stage and then became confused and disorientated saying that she could not breathe and was going to die. Immediately following this she collapsed.

## Examination

The woman is unconscious and unrouseable to painful stimuli. The blood pressure is 98/40 mmHg and heart rate 120/min. The oxygen saturation is 86 per cent on air and respiratory rate 20/min. The heart sounds are normal but on chest examination there are inspiratory crackles throughout the chest.

The abdomen is soft with intermittent contractions continuing, and in fact the fetal head is now visible at the perineum. There is no vaginal bleeding.

## Questions
- What is the likely diagnosis and differential diagnosis?
- How would you manage this woman?

## ANSWER 76

The diagnosis is likely to be an amniotic fluid embolism.

Differential diagnoses include:

- pulmonary embolism
- myocardial infarction
- vasovagal attack.

The factors leading to the diagnosis of amniotic fluid embolism rather than one of the differentials are the history of sudden collapse without preceding chest pain, and the fact that this occurred around the time of rupture of membranes. Amniotic fluid embolism is also often preceded by premonitory symptoms, restlessness, confusion or cyanosis. A vasovagal attack is very unlikely as this is usually associated with bradycardia and would not account for the chest signs or decreased oxygen saturation.

Amniotic fluid embolism occurs when amniotic fluid enters the maternal circulation. This is usually during labour but can occur with maternal trauma or very occasionally after delivery. It is rare (five cases in the last Confidential Enquiry into Maternal and Child Health 2000–2002), unpredictable, sudden and commonly fatal. Women who die tend to do so within an hour or so of becoming unwell, having developed acute hypoxia, coagulopathy and cardiac arrest.

### Management

The baby should be delivered immediately as this will facilitate more effective resuscitation of the mother. In this case a simple forceps delivery should be performed. If the baby was not deliverable vaginally then immediate Caesarean section should be performed. Massive postpartum haemorrhage is very likely and syntocinon infusion should be commenced with further postpartum haemorrhage strategies such as ergometrine, carboprost, embolization or hysterectomy anticipated.

---

**!** | **Resuscitation of the mother after suspected amniotic fluid embolism**

- Insertion of two large-bore intravenous cannulae
- Request for full blood count, urea and electrolytes, clotting profile, fibrin-degradation products
- Crossmatch 6 units blood and have platelets and fresh-frozen plasma available
- 100 per cent oxygen by bag and mask initially with intubation by the anaesthetist as soon as possible
- Volume expansion with colloid fluids
- Transfer to intensive care unit as soon as possible

---

 KEY POINTS

- Sudden collapse in labour is an obstetric emergency.
- The diagnosis of amniotic fluid embolism is usually made postmortem.

## CASE 77: POSTPARTUM BLEEDING

### History
A 32-year-old woman is brought into the delivery suite by ambulance 6 days following a vaginal delivery at 39 weeks' gestation. The pregnancy and labour had been unremarkable and the placenta was delivered by controlled cord traction.

Following delivery the woman had been discharged home after 6 h. She reported that the lochia had been heavy for the first 2 days but that it had then settled to less than a period. However today she had suddenly felt crampy abdominal pain and felt a gush of fluid, followed by very heavy bleeding. The blood has soaked through clothes and she had passed large clots, which she describes as the size of her fist. She feels dizzy when she stands up and is nauseated.

### Examination
She is pale with cool and clammy extremities. She is also drowsy. Her blood pressure is 105/50 mmHg and heart rate is 112/min. On abdominal palpation there is minimal tenderness but the uterus is palpable approximately 6 cm above the symphysis pubis.

Speculum examination reveals large clots of blood in the vagina. When these are removed, the cervix is seen to be open.

### Questions
- What is the diagnosis?
- What is your immediate and subsequent management?
- Should an ultrasound scan be requested?

# ANSWER 77

The diagnosis is secondary postpartum haemorrhage.

---

**!  Postpartum haemorrhage**

Postpartum haemorrhage is defined as the loss of more than 500 mL of blood vaginally following delivery. Primary postpartum haemorrhage is within 24 h. Secondary postpartum haemorrhage occurs between 24 h and 6 weeks following delivery.

---

**!  Common causes of postpartum haemorrhage**

- Retained placental tissue
- Vaginal trauma
- Endometrial infection
- Coagulopathy (e.g. following placental abruption)
- Uterine atony

---

**Immediate management**

This woman is in hypovolaemic shock and needs immediate resuscitation. Two wide-bore cannulae should be inserted and blood sent for full blood count, urea and electrolytes, clotting and crossmatch of 4 units, with further red cells, platelets or fresh-frozen plasma requested depending on further evaluation and blood results.

Immediate intravenous fluid should be administered, usually colloid as volume expansion to maintain cardiac output.

The uterus should be rubbed suprapubically, and if this fails then bimanually, pending administration of 500 μg ergometrine and commencing a syntocinon infusion. These measures stem the blood loss and aid immediate resuscitation while the diagnosis is investigated.

A urinary catheter should be inserted to allow close fluid balance monitoring and renal function.

The anaesthetist and senior obstetrician should be called urgently.

**Subsequent management**

The fact that the cervix is open is pathognomonic of retained tissue, and evacuation of retained products of conception should be arranged once the woman has been resuscitated and blood is available.

In view of the haemodynamic instability, general anaesthetic is preferred.

Intravenous antibiotics should be given.

The woman should be monitored initially in a high-dependency setting until clinically and haematologically stable.

Although she is likely to have had a coagulopathy at admission, she is still at high risk of venous thromboembolism as she is probably septic, postpartum and has undergone anaesthetic. Thromboembolic stockings and heparin should therefore be administered postoperatively.

**Ultrasound scan**

Ultrasound scan would not be indicated in this scenario. First, an open cervix implies retained products and it would therefore be superfluous. Second, an examination under anaesthetic is warranted anyway to establish any other cause of bleeding, such as vaginal or perineal trauma. Third, retained products may be confused with blood clot on post-partum ultrasound.

 **KEY POINTS**

- Postpartum women with retained products of conception become very ill very quickly. Once the diagnosis is made they need intravenous antibiotics and urgent evacuation of the uterus.

# CASE 78: LABOUR

## History

A 31-year-old woman is admitted with contractions at 40 weeks' gestation. This is her fourth pregnancy, having had two terminations approximately 10 years ago and an elective Caesarean section for breech presentation 3 years ago.

During this pregnancy she has had an amniocentesis because of a high estimated risk for Down's syndrome at 11–14-week scan. However a normal karyotype was found and subsequent fetal echocardiography was normal. In view of her previous Caesarean section she was seen by the obstetric consultant in the antenatal clinic at 28 weeks to discuss mode of delivery. After counselling, a plan was agreed for a vaginal delivery.

She was admitted with spontaneous rupture of membranes after which she had begun to contract irregularly. The contractions became stronger and more regular over the next 2 h after admission and she requested an epidural. Vaginal examination was performed and the cervix was found to be 4 cm dilated. The head was in the occipito transverse position, 1 cm above the level of the ischial spines. There was a small amount of caput and moulding.

An epidural was sited and an indwelling urinary catheter inserted. Three hours later the woman reported more severe pain which did not disappear between contractions. At that time approximately 200 mL of fresh blood was seen coming from the vagina.

## Examination

The heart rate is 105/min and blood pressure 105/58 mmHg. The woman feels warm and well perfused. The abdomen is soft and the uterus is also soft but very tender, with easy palpation of fetal parts. On vaginal examination the cervix is 6 cm dilated and the fetal head feels high in the pelvis and poorly applied to the cervix. The catheter contains blood-stained urine.

---

 **INVESTIGATIONS**

The cardiotocograph (CTG) is described below and shown in Fig. 78.1.

*CTG report*:
Fetal heart rate initially 150/min with variability 20/min
Sudden prolonged fall in fetal heart rate to 80/min
No accelerations
Loss of uterine activity at time of fetal bradycardia

---

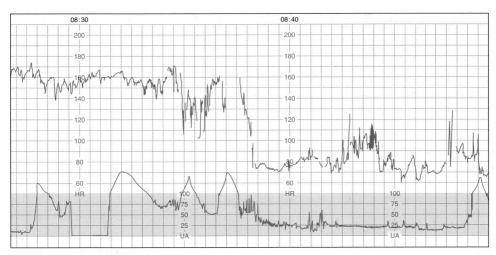

**Figure 78.1** Cardiotocograph.

## Questions

- What is the likely diagnosis?
- How would you manage this patient?
- What are the possible further complications in this patient?

# ANSWER 78

The CTG shows that the contractions have stopped. This can be due to the pressure transducer losing contact with the patient, but in this case the combination of other factors and the fact that the uterus is soft on palpation suggests that the contractions really have suddenly stopped.

The diagnosis is of uterine rupture. The constant pain, vaginal bleeding, sudden loss of contractions, change in CTG, easy palpation of fetal parts and haematuria are all classic features. Uterine rupture is thought to occur in up to 1 in 200 labours following Caesarean section. It is more common when labour is induced with prostaglandins or augmented with oxytocin infusion, but may occur even in an apparently 'normal' labour such as this. Uterine rupture may very rarely occur in women without previous Caesarean section, either because of previous surgery such as myomectomy, with trauma, or spontaneously. The major risk factor for uterine rupture is previous Caesarean section.

General resuscitation measures should be commenced immediately:

- large-bore intravenous access
- full blood count, coagulation test
- 6 unit crossmatch requested
- intravenous fluids.

The emergency theatre team, senior obstetrician and paediatrician should be summoned and the woman transferred to theatre immediately for laparotomy, which may need to be under general anaesthetic as the epidural is unlikely to be adequate for laparotomy within a few minutes.

At laparotomy, the fetus should be delivered from the abdomen and the placenta removed. It may be possible to repair the uterine defect. However, if bleeding is substantial then other measures may need to be employed such as a B-Lynch haemostatic suture or even hysterectomy.

If the uterus is preserved, then any future pregnancies should be very closely monitored with elective delivery by Caesarean section at 37 weeks' gestation.

---

**!** | **Complications of uterine rupture**

- *Fetal*:
  - death
  - cerebral palsy from hypoxic brain injury
- *Maternal*:
  - postpartum haemorrhage
  - hysterectomy
  - coagulopathy

---

**KEY POINTS**

- Dehiscence of a previous Caesarean section scar can range from a dramatic to subtle presentation.
- Change in CTG pattern, persistent abdominal pain cessation of contractions, maternal tachycardia or haematuria should alert the clinician to the possibility of rupture.

# CASE 79: LABOUR

## History

A midwife is concerned about a cardiotocograph (CTG) on the labour ward. The woman is 42 years old and had an elective Caesarean section 3 years ago for twins. After counselling, she decided to opt for a vaginal delivery in this pregnancy. She is now 38 weeks 1 day's gestation and presented to the labour ward an hour ago. She was found to have contractions, three in 10 min lasting 50 s each. There was no reported rupture of membranes.

At the time of arrival, examination revealed a symphysiofundal height of 39 cm, cephalic presentation and 3/5 palpable abdominally. Vaginal examination revealed intact membranes with the head 1 cm above the ischial spines, occipitoanterior position and the cervix 5 cm dilated.

She was commenced on continuous CTG monitoring (because of the previous Caesarean section), which showed an initial baseline rate of 135/min, good variability, accelerations and no decelerations.

Twenty minutes ago spontaneous rupture of membranes occurred with clear liquor leaking.

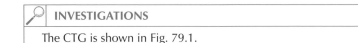

| INVESTIGATIONS |
| --- |
| The CTG is shown in Fig. 79.1. |

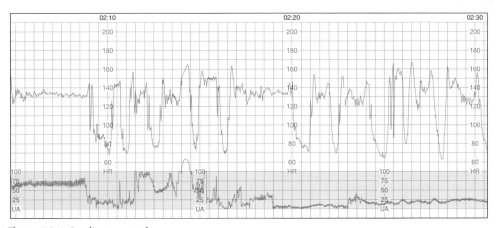

**Figure 79.1** Cardiotocograph.

## Questions
- Describe and classify the CTG.
- What are the possible causes for this CTG pattern?
- What should be your subsequent management?

# ANSWER 79

The CTG shows a baseline rate of 130/min and variability of 15/min. There are variable decelerations to approximately 70/min lasting 30–90 s. Although there are no normal accelerations there is 'shouldering' before and after the decelerations, a sign of the fetus increasing its heart rate in response to the increased blood flow after the deceleration.

This CTG is unsatisfactory because the tocometer is not registering contractions.

 **Definition of variable decelerations**

Decelerations that vary in shape, size and timing

The presence of variable decelerations with no other suspicious features leads to the classification of this CTG as non-reassuring.

## Management

In this situation, the recent history of spontaneous rupture of membranes indicates immediate vaginal assessment to rule out cord prolapse as the cause of the suddenly abnormal CTG. This would be a classic presentation for cord prolapse, though the condition itself is very rare.

Much more commonly variable decelerations are caused by cord compression (by the uterine wall or, for example, by the fetal hand)

If, as is normally the case, the cord is not palpable and the baby is not easily deliverable by instrumental delivery, then further assessment of fetal wellbeing is required as the abnormality of the CTG has already lasted 20 min. This should be by fetal blood sampling (FBS).

In this case FBS gave the following result:
pH: 7.23
Base excess: −4.0 mmol/L

With a pH between 7.20 and 7.25, it is reasonable to manage the woman expectantly and repeat the FBS in 30 min. This was done and the second result was:
pH: 7.22
Base excess: −5.1 mmol/L

At this stage the woman was fully dilated and pushing involuntarily, and the baby was delivered spontaneously soon after the sample was taken.

In this case the fetal blood pH was relatively reassuring despite the dramatic appearance of the CTG. It is possible to avoid Caesarean section in such cases with appropriate use of FBS. It should be remembered that FBS is contraindicated in certain conditions such as maternal HIV, hepatitis or potential fetal-bleeding disorders.

---

🔑 **KEY POINTS**

- CTGs are classified according to national guidelines (as shown in Tables 79.1 and 79.2).
- FBS can often confirm fetal wellbeing despite a non-reassuring or abnormal CTG, and thus avoid an unnecessary operative delivery.

---

**Table 79.1 Classification of fetal heart rate traces according to national guidelines on electronic fetal monitoring**

| Category | Definition |
| --- | --- |
| Normal | A CTG where all four features fall into the reassuring category |
| Suspicious | A CTG whose features fall into one of the non-reassuring categories and the remainder of the features are reassuring |
| Pathological | A CTG whose features fall into two or more non-reassuring categories or one or more abnormal categories |

Reproduced with permission from Royal College of Obstetricians and Gynaecologists. *The use of Electronic Fetal Monitoring: the use and interpretation of cardiotocography in intrapartum fetal surveillance.* Evidence-based Clinical Guideline Number 8. London: Royal College of Obstetricians and Gynaecologists, 2001

**Table 79.2 Classification of fetal heart rate features according to national guidelines on electronic fetal monitoring**

| Feature | Baseline (beats/min) | Variability (beats/min) | Decelerations | Accelerations |
| --- | --- | --- | --- | --- |
| Reassuring | 110–160 | ⩾5 | None | Present |
| Non-reassuring | 100–109; 161–180 | <5 for >40 to <90 min | Early deceleration; variable deceleration; single prolonged deceleration up to 3 min | The absence of accelerations with an otherwise normal CTG are of uncertain significance |
| Abnormal | <100; >180; sinusoidal pattern ⩾10 min | | Atypical variable decelerations; late decelerations; single prolonged deceleration >3 min | |

Reproduced with permission from Royal College of Obstetricians and Gynaecologists. *The use of Electronic Fetal Monitoring: the use and interpretation of cardiotocography in intrapartum fetal surveillance.* Evidence-based Clinical Guideline Number 8. London: Royal College of Obstetricians and Gynaecologists, 2001

# CASE 80: LABOUR

## History

A 22-year-old woman in her second pregnancy has arrived on the labour ward at 38 weeks 3 days. She had a normal delivery 18 months ago. This pregnancy has been complicated by persistent vomiting until 20 weeks, and more recently by anaemia. She reports contractions commencing approximately 4 h ago. She took paracetamol at home and tried to relieve the pain with a bath, but now feels she cannot cope with the pain.

She had a show 2 days ago but has had no bleeding since then and has not noticed any vaginal leak. She has felt the baby moving normally all day.

## Examination

The blood pressure is 110/58 mmHg and heart rate is 98/min. The presentation is cephalic with 2/5 palpable abdominally. Uterine contractions are palpable and the uterus is non-irritable. On vaginal examination the cervix is 5 cm dilated and the head is 1 cm above the ischial spines. The fetus is right occipitotransverse with mild caput and moulding. The membranes are intact but rupture spontaneously during examination, with clear liquor draining.

The woman requests an epidural for pain relief and is therefore commenced on continuous cardiotocograph monitoring. After 20 min you are called in to review the situation.

---

| 🔍 | INVESTIGATIONS |
|---|---|
| | The CTG as you walk in is shown in Fig. 80.1. |

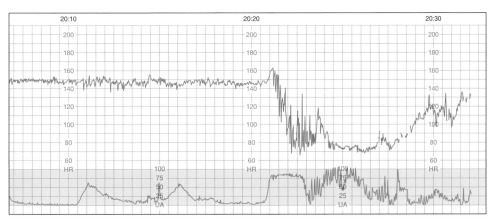

**Figure 80.1** Cardiotocograph.

## Questions
- Describe the CTG.
- What are the possible causes of this CTG?
- What management would be appropriate now?

## ANSWER 80

### CTG interpretation

The initial 15 min of CTG shows a baseline of 145/min with normal variability (12/min) and no visible acceleration or decelerations. Following this there is a drop in fetal heart rate to 70/min for 7 min before gradual recovery to 125/min. Contractions are 2 in 10 until the tocograph becomes unreadable.

This is a previously low-risk pregnancy and this CTG shows a fetal bradycardia (reduction in baseline heart rate to below 100/min). In many cases no cause is identified.

---

**!**  **Causes of fetal bradycardia**

- Placental abruption
- Uterine rupture
- Maternal hypotension (e.g. after epidural insertion)
- Bleeding vasa praevia

---

### Management

If a bradycardia continues for more than 5 min, plans should be made to deliver immediately by 'crash' Caesarean section under general anaesthetic. The labour ward theatre team should be called (including anaesthetist, obstetric registrar, paediatrician, midwife in charge, theatre staff) and the woman transferred to the operating theatre. On occasion the bradycardia recovers as preparation is underway for the Caesarean, in which case the plan may be reviewed. Otherwise the baby should be delivered immediately.

In this case the bradycardia did not recover and the baby was delivered within 12 min of the decision being made. No cause was found for the bradycardia at Caesarean section.

---

**INVESTIGATIONS**

The umbilical artery cord blood analysis at delivery was:

|  | Artery | Vein |
|---|---|---|
| pH | 7.06 | 7.23 |
| $pCO_2$ | 8.20 mmHg | 6.30 mmHg |
| Base excess | −6.4 mmol/L | −5.2 mmol/L |

---

The baby initially made poor respiratory effort and had a heart rate less than 100/min, but recovered quickly with drying and warming. The Apgar score for the baby was 5 at 1 min and 9 at 5 min.

---

  **KEY POINTS**

- Fetal bradycardia persisting for more than 5 min necessitates immediate delivery.
- There is no place for a fetal blood sample in the management of fetal bradycardia.
- A cause is not always found for an abnormal CTG.

---

# CASE 81: PAIN AND FEVER IN PREGNANCY

## History

A woman aged 26 years is referred by her general practitioner. She is 36 weeks' gestation in her fourth pregnancy, having had one miscarriage and two term vaginal deliveries.

In this pregnancy she has been seen twice in the day assessment unit, the first time at 31 weeks for an episode of vaginal bleeding for which no cause was attributed. The second time was at 35 weeks after she awoke with damp bed sheets. No liquor had been detected on speculum examination at the time and she was discharged. For the last 2 days she has been feeling generally unwell with a fever, decreased appetite and a headache as well as abdominal discomfort. She reports the baby moving less than normal for the last few days, with approximately 8–10 movements per day.

She has not noticed any vaginal bleeding but her discharge has been more than normal and there is an offensive odour to it.

## Examination

Her temperature is 37.8°C, blood pressure 106/68 mmHg and heart rate 109/min. On abdominal palpation symphysiofundal height is 34 cm and the fetus is cephalic with 3/5 palpable. There is generalized uterine tenderness and irritability. On speculum examination the cervix is closed and a green/grey discharge is seen within the vagina.

---

### 🔍 INVESTIGATIONS

|  |  | Normal range for pregnancy |
|---|---|---|
| Haemoglobin | 10.9 g/dL | 11–14 g/dL |
| Mean cell volume | 80 fL | 74.4–95.6 fL |
| White cell count | $17.3 \times 10^9$/L | $6–16 \times 10^9$/L |
| Platelets | $327 \times 10^9$/L | $150–400 \times 10^9$/L |
| C-reactive protein | 68 mg/L | <5 mg/L |

The cardiotocograph (CTG) is shown in Fig. 81.1.

---

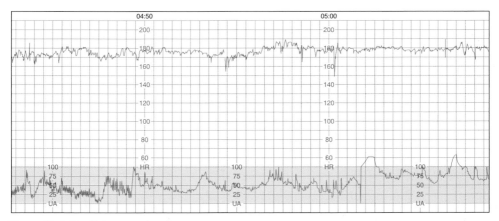

Figure 81.1 Cardiotocograph.

## Questions

- What is the diagnosis?
- How should this woman be managed?

# ANSWER 81

The diagnosis is of chorioamnionitis secondary to prolonged preterm rupture of membranes. Although spontaneous rupture of membranes was not confirmed at the previous attendance at 35 weeks, it seems probable that in fact this did occur at that time. Ascending organisms have thus colonized the uterus and resulted in infection. The result is a maternal systemic reaction causing her symptoms: tachycardia, tenderness, leucocytosis, and raised C-reactive protein.

The fetus is also affected as shown by the fetal tachycardia.

Chorioamnionitis is a significant cause of both fetal and maternal morbidity and mortality, and should be treated as an obstetric emergency.

Management should be instigated immediately. Initial microbial specimens should be obtained from high vaginal swab and maternal blood cultures.

Intravenous broad-spectrum antibiotic should be commenced to cover both anaerobic and aerobic organisms. Intravenous fluids should be commenced to counter the effects of vasodilatation and pyrexia, and because the woman is unable to drink adequately. Paracetamol should be given regularly for the pyrexia and abdominal discomfort.

The baby needs delivery by induction of labour – women with chorioamnionitis often labour rapidly. Risks of Caesarean section in the presence of infection are significant in terms of bleeding, uterine atony and disseminated intravascular coagulopathy. However continuous CTG should be employed and immediate Caesarean section performed if it deteriorates.

Steroids (to prevent potential respiratory distress syndrome) are contraindicated in this woman as they may increase the severity of infection.

After delivery, the baby will need to be reviewed by the paediatrician and given a septic screen and course of intravenous antibiotics.

---

 **KEY POINTS**

- Chorioamnionitis is a significant cause of fetal and maternal morbidity and must be managed aggressively with antibiotics and induction of labour.
- An uncomplicated fetal tachycardia should be managed with fluids and paracetamol to the mother, with antibiotics if infection is suspected.
- Delivery should be expedited if any more suspicious CTG features develop.

## CASE 82: HEADACHE IN PREGNANCY

### History
A 32-year-old woman who is 34 weeks' gestation has felt generally unwell for 24 h. She has a headache and has noticed odd visual symptoms such as 'wobbling' of objects. She initially felt that she had a viral infection but the symptoms are worsening and she thought she should get 'checked out'.

She has epigastric discomfort and nausea. Her legs have been swollen for some weeks but now her hands and face are puffy. The baby has been moving normally and there is no lower abdominal pain and no bleeding or abnormal discharge.

She booked in the pregnancy at 10 weeks with a blood pressure of 107/60 mmHg. Booking blood tests and 12- and 20-week ultrasound scans were normal.

### Examination
Her blood pressure is 140/85 mmHg and pulse rate 98/min. There is moderate oedema to the knees and she also appears digitally and facially oedematous. The fundi are normal.

On abdominal palpation there is mild right upper quadrant and epigastric tenderness. The uterus is not tender and symphysiofundal height measures 33 cm. The fetus is cephalic and free, with fetal parts easily felt on palpation. Patellar reflexes are normal.

---

### INVESTIGATIONS

| | | Normal range for pregnancy |
|---|---|---|
| Haemoglobin | 9.3 g/dL | 11–14 g/dL |
| Packed cell volume | 42% | 31–38% |
| Mean cell volume | 81 fL | 74.4–95.6 fL |
| White cell count | $6.0 \times 10^9$/L | $6–16 \times 10^9$/L |
| Platelets | $97 \times 10^9$/L | $150–400 \times 10^9$/L |
| Sodium | 139 mmol/L | 130–140 mmol/L |
| Potassium | 4.2 mmol/L | 3.3–4.1 mmol/L |
| Urea | 4 mmol/L | 2.4–4.3 mmol/L |
| Creatinine | 83 µmol/L | 34–82 µmol/L |
| Alanine transaminase | 172 IU/L | 6–32 IU/L |
| Alkaline phosphatase | 238 IU/L | 30–300 IU/L |
| Gamma glutamyl transaminase | 26 IU/L | 5–43 IU/L |
| Bilirubin | 37 µmol/L | 3–14 µmol/L |
| Albumin | 26 g/dL | 28–37 g/L |
| Urate | 0.38 mmol/L | 0.14–0.38 mmol/L |
| Urinalysis: + protein | | |

---

### Questions
- What is the likely diagnosis?
- How would you further investigate and manage this patient?

# ANSWER 82

The diagnosis is HELLP syndrome (haemolysis, elevated liver enzymes and low platelets).

HELLP syndrome is part of the spectrum of pre-eclampsia, and is a serious condition with a relatively high maternal mortality (1 per cent) and perinatal mortality (up to 60 per cent). Maternal complications include placental abruption, renal failure, liver failure and disseminated intravascular coagulopathy (DIC). Fetal complications arise from prematurity, abruption and uteroplacental insufficiency.

The diagnosis is made on the blood test results showing the relevant features of HELLP. In this case there is also pregnancy-induced hypertension and proteinuria. However these clinical features do not need to be present to make the diagnosis of HELLP syndrome.

HELLP may present antenatally or in the first few days postpartum.

The symptom of epigastric or right upper quadrant pain should always raise suspicion in a pregnant woman, as it is a sign of liver capsule stretching and may precede liver rupture.

## Investigation and management
The woman needs urgent delivery. This may be vaginal, with regular monitoring of the blood test results and proteinuria every 6 h. Hourly blood pressure should be recorded.

A clotting screen is helpful to indicate any severe risk of bleeding at delivery. If the cervix is unfavourable and the woman is nulliparous then Caesarean section may be considered, but the increased risk of associated bleeding should be borne in mind.

Fetal wellbeing should be checked with cardiotocography and possibly ultrasound for growth, liquor volume and umbilical artery Doppler. The fetal parts being easily palpable may be suggestive of oligohydramnios from uteroplacental insufficiency.

Steroids should be administered to reduce the chance of respiratory distress syndrome, though there may be insufficient time before delivery for them to the effective.

Postnatally the woman should be monitored in hospital for up to 5 days as the condition may deteriorate before recovery. Once recovery occurs it is usually complete, but there is an increased risk of pre-eclampsia (and possibly HELLP syndrome) in subsequent pregnancies.

---

 KEY POINTS

- HELLP syndrome is a very serious condition and requires urgent delivery.

---

# CASE 83: PROLONGED PREGNANCY

## History

A 23-year-old primigravid woman is seen by the midwife in the antenatal clinic at 41 weeks' gestation. She had an ultrasound scan at 12 weeks that was consistent with her menstrual dates. At 28 weeks she developed pelvic pain and a diagnosis of symphysio-pelvic dysfunction (SPD) was made. She has had regular physiotherapy and needs to use a stick to walk on most days. She has been otherwise well in the pregnancy and all blood tests have been within the normal range. She reports normal fetal movements. There is no reported vaginal loss.

## Examination

Her blood pressure is 126/72 mmHg. The symphysiofundal height is 40 cm and the presentation is cephalic, 2/5 palpable. Subjectively the liquor volume feels normal.

You note that she appears unhappy, and on questioning she says that she is just very uncomfortable as a result of the SPD.

|  INVESTIGATIONS |
| --- |
| Urinalysis: negative |

## Question

• Explain the appropriate management for this woman from now.

# ANSWER 83

The estimated due date is only a guide and women are expected to deliver between 3 weeks before and 2 weeks after this date. Twenty-five per cent of women will not have delivered by 41 weeks (18 per cent by 42 weeks). As this woman is 41 weeks, plans should be made for induction of labour if spontaneous labour does not occur in the next few days.

## Cervical sweep

A cervical sweep involves a vaginal examination to assess the cervix, and insertion of the finger through the cervical os if possible and then sweeping it around the inside of the lower uterus, trying to separate the membranes from the cervix. Such membrane sweeping decreases the rate of prolonged pregnancy (>42 weeks).

## Induction of labour

Admission should be planned for induction of labour between 41 and 42 weeks, assuming spontaneous labour has not occurred. This gestation is used because stillbirth increases with gestational age above 37 weeks. There is a similar increase in neonatal mortality.

| ! Stillbirth rate according to gestation |
|---|
| • 1 per 3000 births at 37 weeks |
| • 2 per 3000 births at 42 weeks |
| • 3 per 3000 births at 43 weeks |

Although the woman is in some discomfort, early induction should be avoided as far as possible, as success of induction increases with gestation.

## Method of induction of labour

Prostaglandins should be used for induction of labour with insertion of prostaglandin gel (or pessary) into the posterior fornix of the vagina. The fetus should be monitored by cardiotocograph for 20 min before and after as prostaglandins may cause uterine hyperstimulation and fetal distress.

If spontaneous contractions have not started or membranes ruptured after 6 h, then the prostaglandin should be repeated. If contractions have commenced (regardless of whether membranes are intact) then vaginal examination should be repeated every 4 h.

If membrane rupture has occurred but contractions have not started after 2–4 h, then an oxytocin infusion would normally be commenced. Subsequent management is as for normal labour.

## Expectant management beyond 42 weeks

If the woman declines induction of labour by 42 weeks, fetal wellbeing should be assessed with ultrasound for fetal growth and liquor volume. Fetal movements should be monitored, with induction regularly reconsidered.

---

 KEY POINTS

- Perinatal mortality and morbidity increase with advancing gestational age, and induction of labour is therefore recommended between 41 and 42 weeks' gestation.
- Prostaglandins are the main drugs used for induction, and repeated administrations may be necessary.

## CASE 84: PAIN IN PREGNANCY

### History

A 28-year-old woman nulliparous woman is admitted to the labour ward at 31 weeks and 6 days' gestation, with abdominal pain.

In this pregnancy she has had chronic low back pain for which she has been under the physiotherapist. She has also been treated for confirmed urinary tract infections on two occasions. She underwent two large-loop excisions of the transformation zone (LLETZ) procedures some years ago. Since then her smears have been normal, the most recent being 10 months ago.

Yesterday she noticed an increase in her discharge with some dark vaginal bleeding and abdominal discomfort. She thought the symptoms may have related to something she had eaten but she now feels intermittent abdominal pain every few minutes, with no pain in between episodes. Fetal movements are normal.

There is no history of leaking of liquor. She has urinary frequency, though this has not worsened recently. She is always constipated.

### Examination

The woman is apyrexial with blood pressure 109/60 mmHg and heart rate 96/min. Symphysiofundal height is 30 cm and moderate contractions are palpated lasting approximately 35 s. The fetus is breech on palpation and the presenting part feels engaged.

No liquor is visible on speculum examination. On vaginal examination the cervix is effaced and 3 cm dilated, with the breech felt −2 cm above the ischial spines and membranes intact.

| INVESTIGATIONS |
| --- |
| *Cardiotocograph (CTG):* |
| Baseline rate 145/min, variability normal (15/min) |
| Accelerations present |
| No decelerations observed |
| Uterine activity recorded 3 in 10 |

### Questions
- What is the diagnosis?
- What factors predispose to this?
- How would you manage this woman?

# ANSWER 84

The woman is in premature labour – she has regular painful contractions (as confirmed by the history, palpation and uterine activity demonstrated on CTG) and the cervix is effaced and dilated.

In this history the possible risk factors are the LLETZ procedures and urinary tract infections, raising the possibility that she could be in premature labour due to a further untreated urinary tract infection. However, many women in premature labour have no obvious risk factors.

> **!** **Risk factors for premature labour**
>
> - *Maternal:*
>   - history of premature delivery
>   - young maternal age
>   - illegal drug use and smoking
>   - chorioamnionitis
>   - pre-eclampsia
>   - polyhydramnios
>   - sepsis
>   - previous cervical surgery/cervical incompetence
> - *Fetal:*
>   - intrauterine growth retardation
>   - congenital abnormality
>   - multiple pregnancy

## Management

- Prevention of respiratory distress syndrome (RDS):
  - antenatal corticosteroids (usually betamethasone intramuscular) prior to delivery reduce the incidence of RDS in premature infants, and ideally two doses should be administered 12 h apart prior to delivery.
  - tocolysis (with atosiban, a beta-agonist or nifedipine) should be started immediately to try and delay labour in order for the steroids to be maximally effective (24 h), and then discontinued. The other indication for tocolysis is to settle contractions long enough for in utero transfer of the mother to a unit with facilities to care for a 31-week baby. In other situations tocolysis does not seem to improve fetal outcome, even though it may prolong time to delivery.
- *Mode of delivery:* although there is evidence that full-term singleton breech babies should be delivered by Caesarean section (rather than vaginally), there is no clear evidence that this applies to preterm infants, and as premature delivery is generally reasonably quick, vaginal delivery should be considered. The contraindications to this would be signs of fetal compromise on CTG, or maternal objection.
- *Postnatal care:* the paediatric team should be informed of any woman in actual or threatened preterm labour, in order that appropriate arrangements are made for care of the infant after delivery.

>  **KEY POINTS**
>
> - Premature delivery is the major cause of perinatal mortality.
> - If a woman goes into premature labour one must consider prevention of RDS and mode of delivery.

# CASE 85: DELIVERY

### History

You are urgently called to the delivery room of a 26-year-old woman to help deliver the baby. The mother is 41 weeks into her second pregnancy, having had a normal term delivery of a 3.97 kg female infant 2 years ago.

Nuchal and anomaly scans were normal and antenatal care was unremarkable. The baby was moving normally prior to labour.

When she arrived on labour ward contracting, the symphysiofundal height was noted to be 41 cm.

At first assessment the cervix was 3 cm dilated and she was advised to continue mobilizing. Spontaneous rupture of membranes occurred and she was examined again after 4 h and the cervix was still 3 cm. A syntocinon infusion was commenced to augment labour and an epidural sited, with cardiotocograph monitoring also commenced. After 4 h, the cervix was 7 cm and then 10 cm after a further 4 h. The woman was encouraged to start active pushing and 35 min later the head had crowned in a direct occipitoanterior position.

The midwife noticed that the head did not extend normally on the perineum and that the chin appeared to be wedged against the perineum. She had attempted delivery of the shoulders with the next two contractions but this had not been achieved.

### Questions
- What is the diagnosis?
- How would you manage this scenario?

# ANSWER 85

This condition, where the fetal shoulders and trunk fail to deliver after the head, is shoulder dystocia. Complications include perinatal mortality, hypoxic encephalopathy, brachial plexus injury (e.g. Erb's palsy), as well as maternal postpartum haemorrhage and third- or fourth-degree tear.

Shoulder dystocia occurs in 1 in 200 deliveries and is associated with various risk factors (though in many cases it cannot be predicted). In this case the woman had a relatively large previous baby, this baby had persistently been large on examination, she is post dates and progress was a little slow.

| ! | Risk factors for shoulder dystocia |
|---|---|

- Estimated fetal weight >4.5 kg
- Previous big baby (>4 kg)
- Previous shoulder dystocia
- Slow progress in the first and/or second stage of labour
- Post dates delivery

### Management

This is an obstetric emergency and the emergency bell should be activated with help summoned from the senior midwife, other available midwives, anaesthetist and paediatrician, as well as the most senior obstetrician available.

A series of manoeuvres are practiced by labour ward staff at 'skills and drills' sessions in preparation for such an event. These are incorporated into the mnemonic **HELPERR**, which is taken from the Advanced Life Support in Obstetrics (ALSO®) programme. The programme and its copyright are owned by the American Academy of Family Physicians (www.aafp.org/also).

1 *Call for Help.*
2 *Consider Episiotomy:* this will not allow the shoulders to deliver but will allow manipulation of the baby to achieve delivery.
3 *Elevate the Legs* (McRoberts Manoeuvre): the procedure involves flexing the maternal hips, thus positioning the thighs up onto the abdomen. This simulates the squatting position, with the advantage of increasing the inlet diameter.
4 *Suprapubic Pressure:* external manual suprapubic pressure is applied to the fetus' anterior shoulder, in such a way that the shoulder will adduct or collapse anteriorly and encourage the baby's shoulder to pass under the symphysis pubis. Pressure is at first constant for 60 s, and then in a rocking fashion for a further 60 s.
5 *The operator's fingers should Enter the pelvis:* the index and middle fingers should be inserted past the fetal head and behind the anterior shoulder, then pressure exerted on the back of that shoulder to attempt to rotate the baby (Rubin's manoeuvre). This can also be tried with the posterior shoulder from the front of the fetus, rotating the shoulder toward the symphysis in the same direction as with the Rubin II manoeuvre (Wood screw manoeuvre).
6 *Removal of the posterior arm:* the clinician must insert his or her hand far into the vagina and locate the posterior arm. Once the arm is located, the elbow should be flexed so that the forearm may be delivered in a sweeping motion over the anterior chest wall of the fetus.
7 *Roll onto all fours position:* If the above manoeuvres fail, the woman should be Rolled onto the all fours position which increases the true obstetrical conjugate by as much as 10 mm and the sagittal measurement of the pelvic outlet up to 20 mm.

Delivery usually occurs by stage 5. If it fails then last resort measures are the procedure of replacing the fetal head into the pelvis and performing emergency Caesarean section or performing symphysiotomy (if caesarean delivery is not an option) to enlarge the pelvic diameters.

 **KEY POINTS**

- Shoulder dystocia is an obstetric emergency and requires immediate action.
- All health professionals delivering babies must be well rehearsed with the appropriate manoeuvres.

## CASE 86: HEADACHE IN PREGNANCY

### History

A 17-year-old girl is admitted to the labour ward by ambulance because of a severe headache and reduced fetal movements. This is her first pregnancy. She did not discover she was pregnant until very late and was uncertain of her last menstrual period date so was dated by ultrasound scan at 23 weeks. According to that scan she is now 37 weeks.

When she was first booked in the antenatal clinic her blood pressure was 120/68 mmHg and urinalysis negative. The blood pressure was last checked 1 week ago and was 132/74 mmHg and urine was negative again. Booking blood tests were all normal.

This morning she woke with a frontal headache which has persisted despite paracetamol. She says that her vision is a bit blurred but she cannot be more specific about this. She also reports nausea and epigastric discomfort, but has not vomited. She denies leg or finger swelling.

### Examination

The blood pressure is 164/106 mmHg. This is repeated twice at 15 min intervals and is found to be 160/110 mmHg and 164/112 mmHg. She is apyrexial and her heart rate is 83/min. Her face is minimally swollen and fundoscopy is normal. Cardiac and respiratory examinations are normal. Abdominally she is tender in the epigastrium and beneath the right costal margin, but the uterus is soft and non-tender. The fetus is cephalic and 3/5 palpable.

The legs and fingers are mildly oedematous and lower limb reflexes are very brisk, with clonus.

---

**INVESTIGATIONS**

|  |  | *Normal range for pregnancy* |
|---|---|---|
| Haemoglobin | 11.6 g/dL | 11–14 g/dL |
| Packed cell volume | 42.2% | 31–38% |
| Mean cell volume | 79 fL | 74.4–95.6 fL |
| White cell count | 5 × 10⁹/L | 6–16 × 10⁹/L |
| Platelets | 126 × 10⁹/L | 150–400 × 10⁹/L |
| Sodium | 141 mmol/L | 130–140 mmol/L |
| Potassium | 4.0 mmol/L | 3.3–4.1 mmol/L |
| Urea | 3.8 mmol/L | 2.4–4.3 mmol/L |
| Creatinine | 92 μmol/L | 34–82 μmol/L |
| Alanine transaminase | 189 IU/L | 6–32 IU/L |
| Alkaline phosphatase | 74 IU/L | 30–300 IU/L |
| Gamma glutamyl transaminase | 34 IU/L | 5–43 IU/L |
| Bilirubin | 12 μmol/L | 3–14 μmol/L |
| Albumin | 24 g/L | 28–37 g/L |
| Urate | 0.46 mmol/L | 0.14–0.38 mmol/L |

Urinalysis: ++++ protein

*Cardiotocograph (CTG)*: baseline 140/min, reduced variability (5–10/min). Variable decelerations, occasional accelerations.

---

### Questions
- What is the diagnosis?
- How would you manage this patient?

## ANSWER 86

The woman has pre-eclampsia with rapid onset and severity of symptoms and signs suggesting severe or 'fulminant' disease. She is at high risk of developing eclampsia.

The headache and visual disturbance are typical features of cerebral oedema; the right upper quadrant pain of subcapsular liver swelling and the proteinuria occurs from renal involvement.

The blood tests show typical features of severe pre-eclampsia:

- elevated liver transaminases
- elevated urate
- elevated creatinine.

The platelet count is at the lower end of the normal range for pregnancy and if reduced further, with raised bilirubin would suggest development of HELLP syndrome (haemolysis, elevated liver enzymes and low platelets).

### Management

This is an obstetric emergency and the senior midwife, anaesthetist and senior obstetrician should be informed immediately. The only definitive treatment for pre-eclampsia is delivery of the baby, but the maternal status must be stabilized first. In this case she should be admitted and have an intravenous cannula inserted. Blood should be sent for coagulation and for group and save. A urinary catheter should be inserted and fluid input and output carefully monitored for oliguria as a sign of impending renal failure.

In pre-eclampsia although the extracellular fluid is increased (third space), the intravascular volume is generally depleted, so fluid input should be managed carefully with the help of an anaesthetist, balancing adequate renal perfusion with the risk of overload and pulmonary oedema. Where the urine output is decreased, a central venous line may be needed for more accurate assessment of volume status.

The woman should be given an antihypertensive to reduce her blood pressure (thus reducing the risk of cerebral haemorrhage). If initial oral antihypertensives are not effective, a titrated intravenous infusion should be used.

Magnesium sulphate infusion reduces the risk of an eclamptic fit in women with severe pre-eclampsia and should be commenced.

The CTG shows reduced variability and occasional variable decelerations. This suggests that the reduced fetal movements may be due to fetal distress, probably from uteroplacental insufficiency. Caesarean section would therefore be the mode of delivery of choice, but only when the maternal blood pressure is under control and the coagulation screen result is available.

Postnatally the condition may not improve for 48 h or more, and the woman should be nursed in a high-dependency setting until the blood pressure is under control, renal output is normal, symptoms have settled and blood results are returning to normal.

---

 **KEY POINTS**

- Pre-eclampsia causes widespread endothelial dysfunction, with effects on all the body systems. Death can occur from cerebral haemorrhage, eclampsia, pulmonary oedema, renal failure or hepatic rupture.
- Immediate stabilization of the mother should precede delivery of the baby.

# CASE 87: LABOUR

## History

A 36-year-old nulliparous woman at term started having uterine tightenings yesterday morning. These were intermittent initially and she managed to cope with a hot bath and paracetamol, but they have now become increasingly painful and frequent. This morning she came in because she had ruptured membranes at home an hour and a half ago. She has continued to notice normal fetal movements.

Since arrival the blood pressure, temperature and heart rate have been within the normal range and the liquor has remained clear. She has been examined several times and the findings of each examination are shown in Table 87.1. After the examination at 14.15 a syntocinon infusion was commenced.

Table 87.1 **Examination findings**

| Time | Contractions | Cervical dilatation | Head descent relative to the ischial spines | Position | Caput | Moulding |
|---|---|---|---|---|---|---|
| 10.30 | 3 in 10 | 3 cm | –3 cm | Left occipitotransverse | + | Nil |
| 14.15 | 2 in 10 | 4 cm | –2 cm | Left occipitotransverse | ++ | Nil |
| Syntocinon infusion commenced | | | | | | |
| 18.20 | 3–4 in 10 | 5 cm | –2 cm | Occipitoposterior | ++ | + |
| 22.15 | 4 in 10 | 6 cm | –2 cm | Occipitoposterior | +++ | ++ |

---

🔍 **INVESTIGATIONS**

The cardiotocograph (CTG) is shown in Fig. 87.1.

---

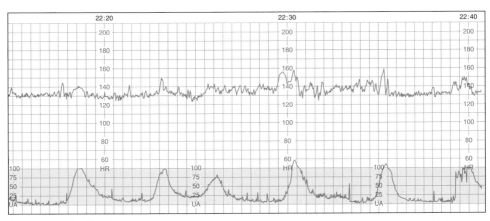

**Figure 87.1** Cardiotocograph.

## Questions

- How do you interpret the examination and CTG findings?
- What factors are associated with this pattern of labour?
- How would you manage this woman?

# ANSWER 87

The examination findings show failure to progress in the first stage in labour. Once labour has been established, the cervix is expected to dilate at approximately 1 cm/h. In this case, despite attempted augmentation with an oxytocic (syntocinon), there has only been 3 cm dilatation in almost 12 h.

This situation is most common in nulliparous women and is termed primary dysfunctional labour. Other associations are malposition (commonly the occipitoposterior position) and increased fetal size (cephalopelvic disproportion).

## Management

Maximum contractions have been achieved (4 in 10 min) with the oxytocic for several hours, and there are increasing signs of obstruction (caput and moulding of the fetal head). In view of this the only management option available is to perform an emergency Caesarean section.

The CTG is normal, but without intervention, the likely scenario is for fetal compromise to occur. Therefore once the decision has been made to proceed with Caesarean section, oxytocin should be discontinued to reduce the effect of the prolonged contractions on the baby. Delivery should be arranged within 30 min of the decision being made.

The important points in arranging delivery by emergency Caesarean section in this case are:

- informed consent, after appropriate explanation, by the mother
- informing the anaesthetist and assistant
- informing the theatre staff and paediatrician
- ranitidine and metoclopramide to the mother (usually intravenous) to minimize gastric aspiration should general anaesthetic be needed
- insertion of an indwelling urinary catheter
- transfer of the woman to theatre, with continuous CTG until delivery.

---

 **KEY POINTS**

- In a primigravid woman the rate of cervical dilatation in normal labour is 1 cm/h.
- Inefficient uterine action must be corrected with syntocinon augmentation before a diagnosis of 'failure to progress' is made.

## CASE 88: POSTPARTUM BLEEDING

### History

A 39-year-old woman in her first pregnancy delivered twin sons 2 h ago. There were no significant antenatal complications. She had been prescribed ferrous sulphate and folic acid during the pregnancy as anaemia prophylaxis, and her last haemoglobin was 10.9 g/dL at 38 weeks.

The fetuses were within normal range for growth and liquor volume on serial scan estimations. A vaginal delivery was planned and she went into spontaneous labour at 38 weeks and 4 days. Due to decelerations in the cardiotocograph (CTG) for the first twin, both babies were delivered by ventouse after 30 min active pushing in the second stage. The midwife recorded both placentae as appearing complete.

As this was a twin pregnancy, an intravenous cannula had been inserted when labour was established and an epidural had been sited. The lochia has been heavy since delivery but the woman is now bleeding very heavily and passing large clots of blood.

On arrival in the room you find that the sheets are soaked with blood and there is also approximately 500 mL of blood clot in a kidney dish on the bed.

### Examination

The woman is conscious but drowsy and pale. The temperature is 35.9°C, blood pressure 120/70 mmHg and heart rate 112/min. The peripheries feel cool. The uterus is palpable to the umbilicus and feels soft. The abdomen is otherwise soft and non-tender. On vaginal inspection there is a second-degree tear which has been sutured but you are unable to assess further due to the presence of profuse bleeding.

The midwife sent blood tests 30 min ago because she was concerned about the blood loss at the time.

| INVESTIGATIONS | | |
|---|---|---|
| | | *Normal range for pregnancy* |
| Haemoglobin | 7.2 g/dL | 11–14 g/dL |
| Mean cell volume | 99.0 fL | 74.4–95.6 fL |
| White cell count | $3.2 \times 10^9$/L | $6–16 \times 10^9$/L |
| Platelets | $131 \times 10^9$/L | $150–400 \times 10^9$/L |
| International normalized ratio (INR) | 1.3 | 0.9–1.2 |
| Activated partial thromboplastin time (APTT) | 39 s | 30–45 s |
| Sodium | 138 mmol/L | 130–140 mmol/L |
| Potassium | 3.5 mmol/L | 3.3–4.1 mmol/L |
| Urea | 5.2 mmol/L | 2.4–4.3 mmol/L |
| Creatinine | 64 μmol/L | 34–82 μmol/L |

### Questions

- What is the diagnosis and what are the likely causes?
- What is the sequence of management options you would employ in this situation?

# ANSWER 88

The diagnosis is primary postpartum haemorrhage (PPH), defined as the loss of more than 500 mL of blood in the first 24 h following delivery. This classification applies even if the blood is lost at Caesarean section or while awaiting placental delivery.

---

**!**  **Causes of and risk factors for postpartum haemorrhage**

- Uterine atony (multiple pregnancy, grand multiparity, polyhydramnios, prolonged labour)
- Antepartum haemorrhage
- Uterine sepsis (chorioamnionitis)
- Retained placenta
- Lower genital tract trauma (perineal or cervical tears)
- Coagulopathy (heparin treatment, inherited bleeding disorders)
- Previous PPH

---

This woman's major risk factor is multiple pregnancy and with the high uterus, the cause is likely to be uterine atony (inability of the uterus to contract adequately). Blood loss is often underestimated, the 'high' uterus may contain a large volume of concealed blood, and the blood pressure in young fit women remains relatively normal until decompensation occurs. Therefore this woman is in fact extremely sick and at risk of cardiac arrest if immediate management is not employed.

The sequence of management strategies is:

- rub up a contraction by placing the dominant hand over the uterus and rubbing and squeezing firmly until the uterus becomes firm
- ensure two large-bore cannulae are inserted with cross-matched blood requested
- recheck full blood count and coagulation
- commence intravenous fluids for volume expansion
- give 500 μg ergometrine intramuscularly or intravenously to enhance uterine contraction
- start a syntocinon infusion to maintain uterine contraction
- consider other uterotonics such as misoprostol or carboprost
- transfer to theatre for examination under anaesthetic to assess for vaginal trauma, cervical laceration or retained placental tissue
- the doctor or midwife should continue bimanual compression until the clinical situation is under control
- if the bleeding does not settle with the above measures then further options are uterine artery embolization or laparotomy with B-Lynch haemostatic suture, uterine artery ligation or hysterectomy.

---

  KEY POINTS

- Uterine compression from the abdomen or bimanually is the first and immediate management strategy for postpartum haemorrhage and should be continued until the clinical situation has settled.
- Clinicians usually underestimate blood loss and in assessing haemodynamic status may forget to take account of concealed loss (into the uterus) and the ability of healthy women to compensate.

---

## CASE 89: LABOUR

### History

A 32-year-old woman presents to the labour ward with abdominal pain. This is her first baby after two miscarriages. She was trying to conceive for 18 months prior to this pregnancy.

Her estimated delivery date was corrected after her 11–14-week scan to make her now 40 weeks and 6 days. All pregnancy blood tests and ultrasound scans have been normal. The baby was breech at 34 weeks but cephalic at 37 weeks.

This morning she had a mucus-like dark-red discharge followed by the onset of irregular period-type pains. Two hours ago she felt a gush of clear fluid from the vagina and since then pains have become much more severe now occurring every 4 min, lasting for 45 s.

The baby has moved normally during the day.

She had a bath at home and took paracetamol but is now distressed and has come to hospital for assessment. Her partner and sister who are both very anxious accompany her.

### Examination

On examination she is comfortable between pains. Her blood pressure is 129/76 mmHg and pulse 101/min. Symphysiofundal height is 37 cm and the fetus is cephalic with 2/5 palpable.

Speculum examination shows clear fluid pooled in the posterior vaginal fornix.

Vaginal examination reveals the cervix to be fully effaced and 4 cm dilated. The position is right occipitoposterior and the head is 2 cm above the ischial spines. There is no fetal caput or moulding.

| INVESTIGATIONS |
| --- |
| Urinalysis: blood ++ |
| Proteinuria: + |
| Leucocytes: negative |
| Nitrites: negative |

### Questions
- What is the diagnosis?
- What is the appropriate management?

# ANSWER 89

This woman is in normal labour.

> **! Definition of labour**
>
> The onset of regular painful contractions with progressive dilatation of the cervix and descent of the presenting part.

Spontaneous rupture of membranes has occurred but is not necessary for the diagnosis of labour.

The woman's observations and examination findings are normal for labour:

- the dark mucus discharge is a 'show' and is not a cause for concern unless the bleeding is fresh or ongoing
- the pulse is almost certainly raised secondarily to the pain
- the haematuria and proteinuria are secondary to contamination by the show and liquor
- the symphysiofundal height is low because the head has descended into the pelvis and because the liquor has been released from the uterus.

## Management

The pregnancy and labour are low risk in that there is no evidence of any fetal or maternal disorder that requires doctor-led care. The woman should therefore remain under midwife-led care and does not need continuous electronic fetal monitoring (cardiotocograph, CTG). The fetus does need assessment for wellbeing with intermittent auscultation for a full minute after a contraction at least every 15 min in the first stage of labour and for a full minute after a contraction every 5 min in the second stage of labour.

> **! Monitoring in low-risk labour**
>
> - Hourly blood pressure
> - Hourly heart rate
> - Four-hourly examinations for cervical dilatation
> - Assessment for meconium

Once labour is established, expected dilatation is approximately 1 cm/h. If this does not occur or if signs suggest that fetal or maternal wellbeing might be compromised, then medical assessment and possible intervention may be indicated.

>  **KEY POINTS**
>
> - Normal labour is the onset of regular painful contractions with progressive dilatation of the cervix and descent of the presenting part.
> - Continuous CTG is not required for low-risk women in normal labour, but intermittent auscultation is essential.

## CASE 90: PAIN IN PREGNANCY

### History

A 35-year-old woman arrives on the labour ward complaining of abdominal pain and vaginal bleeding at 36 weeks 2 days' gestation. The pain started 2 h earlier while she was in a café. She describes constant pain all over her abdomen with exacerbations every few minutes. It is not relieved by lying still or by walking around. The vaginal bleeding is bright red and was initially noticed on the toilet paper and now has stained her under-clothes and trousers. There are no urinary or bowel symptoms.

The baby has been moving normally until today, but the woman has not paid any attention to the movements since the pain started.

This is her first pregnancy and until now progress has been uneventful with shared care between the general practitioner and midwife. Both the 11–14-week and the anomaly scan at 20 weeks were reassuring. Booking and subsequent blood tests were normal. The book-ing blood pressure was 112/68 mmHg and the most recent blood pressure 2 days ago was 128/80 mmHg.

### Examination

She is obviously in significant pain and feels clammy. She is apyrexial, her heart rate is 115/min and blood pressure 110/62 mmHg. The symphysiofundal height is 38 cm and the uterus feels hard and is very tender. It is not possible to feel the presentation of the fetus due to the uterine tightening. On speculum examination there is a trickle of blood through the cervix and the cervix appears closed. Vaginal examination reveals that the cervix is soft and almost full effaced but closed. No fetal heart sounds are heard on auscultation with the hand-held fetal Doppler. Ultrasound scan confirms that the fetus has died.

| INVESTIGATIONS | | |
|---|---|---|
| | | *Normal range for pregnancy* |
| Haemoglobin | 8.1 g/dL | 11–14 g/dL |
| White cell count | 6 × 10⁹/L | 6–16 × 10⁹/L |
| Platelets | 93 × 10⁹/L | 150–400 × 10⁹/L |
| Sodium | 137 mmol/L | 130–140 mmol/L |
| Potassium | 4.0 mmol/L | 3.3–4.1 mmol/L |
| Urea | 6.5 mmol/L | 2.4–4.3 mmol/L |
| Creatinine | 82 µmol/L | 34–82 µmol/L |
| International normalized ratio (INR) | 2.2 | 0.9–1.2 |
| Activated partial thromboplastin time (APTT) | 34 s | 30–45 s |
| D-dimer: positive | | |

### Questions
- What is the diagnosis?
- How do you interpret the examination and blood test findings?
- How would you manage this patient?

# ANSWER 90

The pain and bleeding are due to placental abruption. In this case the presence of vaginal blood classifies it as a 'revealed abruption' but the other signs of hardened 'couvelaire' uterus, raised symphysiofundal height, tachycardia and low haemoglobin all suggest that the major part of the blood is still concealed. This is an extremely important point as the amount of visualized blood can be misleading when there may be 1–2 L of blood within the uterus.

The blood pressure appears normal, but this is because the woman is relatively young and fit – she is able to compensate by increasing heart rate and cardiac output for some time. By the time her blood pressure falls she has decompensated and is critically unwell, so normal blood pressure in young people should always be interpreted carefully. If her blood pressure were checked lying and standing, there would be a significant difference, which would reveal the extent of her hypovolaemia.

The increase in INR, decreased platelets and positive D-dimer test (a reflection of raised fibrin-degradation products) confirm that the woman has developed disseminated intravascular coagulopathy (DIC) as a result of the abruption.

The fetus has died (intrauterine fetal death) because the placenta has separated from the uterus and the uteroplacental circulation has therefore been interrupted.

## Management

This is an obstetric emergency as the woman is hypovolaemic and has developed a coagulopathy. The management centres on correction of the clotting and volume replacement as well as delivery of the baby. The anaesthetist and senior obstetrician should liaise closely in management.

---

**!  Resuscitation of the mother (initial basic procedures)**

- Insertion of two large-bore venous cannulae
- Crossmatch of 6 units of blood
- Request for fresh-frozen plasma and platelets
- Initial fluid resuscitation with intravenous fluids, probably volume expanders
- Insertion of a urinary catheter to monitor urine output

---

As the baby has died there is no indication for Caesarean section, which would put her at risk of further bleeding. Therefore vaginal induction of labour should be initiated. Labour is often rapid after an abruption, and as the cervix is fully effaced and soft it may be sufficient to perform artificial rupture of membranes (ARM) to initiate the process of delivery. At ARM, a large amount of blood is likely to be apparent.

A syntocinon infusion should be commenced immediately after delivery as uterine atony and postpartum haemorrhage are common after significant abruption.

---

**🔑 KEY POINTS**

- Placental abruption is an obstetric emergency and must be aggressively managed as DIC can develop rapidly.
- Placental abruption is commonly associated with the development of pre-eclampsia.
- Labour is usually rapid after abruption, and vaginal delivery poses less risk to the mother than Caesarean section.
- Caesarean section should be reserved for delivering a live but potentially compromised baby.

---

## CASE 91: PERINEAL TEAR

### History

A woman has just delivered her second baby on the labour ward. She is 37 years old and had a previous premature delivery at 34 weeks. In this pregnancy she went into spontaneous labour at 38 weeks after an uncomplicated pregnancy.

The symphysiofundal height was consistent with dates until 37 weeks when the midwife measured it as 41 cm. However, before an ultrasound scan for growth and liquor volume could be arranged the woman went into spontaneous labour.

At the time of admission she was 5 cm dilated and spontaneous rupture of membranes occurred soon after. The baby was delivered 30 min later in the direct occipitoanterior position.

The placenta was delivered by controlled cord traction, after which the midwife noticed a perineal tear. The tear extended from the introitus in the midline and she could see torn muscle fibres suggestive of the torn ends of the external anal sphincter. She has called you to review the patient.

### Questions

- What is the likely diagnosis?
- What factors predispose to this condition?
- How would you manage this patient?

# ANSWER 91

The history suggests a third-degree tear.

> **!  Classification of perineal tears**
>
> - *First degree:* injury to the perineum involving the epithelium or skin but not the perineal muscles
> - *Second degree*: injury to the perineum involving perineal muscles but not involving the anal sphincter
> - *Third degree:* injury to the perineum involving the anal sphincter complex (external anal sphincter (EAS) and internal anal sphincter (IAS)):
>   - 3a: less than 50 per cent of EAS thickness torn
>   - 3b: more than 50 per cent of EAS thickness torn
>   - 3c: IAS torn
> - *Fourth degree*: injury to the perineum involving the anal sphincter complex (EAS and IAS) and rectal mucosa

## Risk factors

Third-degree tears occur in 2–4 per cent of women with the following conditions:

- birthweight over 4 kg
- persistent occipitoposterior position
- nulliparity
- induction of labour
- epidural
- second stage of labour lasting more than 1 h
- episiotomy
- forceps delivery.

Third-degree tear diagnosis depends on the vigilance of the person inspecting a tear and may easily be missed. This has far-reaching consequences, as failure to perform adequate primary repair may increase the chance of longer-term faecal incontinence.

## Management

- The woman should be transferred to theatre for repair. This enables adequate analgesia (spinal or epidural), good exposure, good lighting and availability of appropriate instruments.
- The tear should be repaired in layers:
  - rectal mucosa (if involved)
  - internal anal sphincter (if involved)
  - external anal sphincter
  - perineal muscle
  - vaginal epithelium
  - perineal skin.
- Broad-spectrum antibiotics should be administered to prevent infection from possible contamination by bowel organisms.
- Laxatives should be administered to prevent constipation that might compromise the repair.
- Adequate postoperative analgesia is needed.
- The woman should not generally be discharged until she has opened her bowels.

- A follow-up appointment should be made after approximately 6 weeks to ensure that the woman has no significant bowel symptoms and to refer on to a colorectal specialist if she has.
- Elective Caesarean section should be discussed as a possibility for any subsequent deliveries.

---

 **KEY POINTS**

- Following delivery any vaginal tear must be inspected carefully to ensure that the anal sphincter is not disrupted.
- Any third-degree tears should be repaired in theatre by an experienced operator to avoid future problems with faecal incontinence.

---

# CASE 92: FIT IN PREGNANCY

## History

An obviously pregnant woman is brought to the emergency department having suffered a seizure in the park 20 min ago. She had been alone at the time but the seizure was witnessed by another woman who said that she had stood up from a bench and then suddenly dropped to the ground. She thought she may have hit her head on the side of the bench with the fall. Her arms and legs had been shaking and then were 'stiff and trembling' for about 40 s. The woman's face had gone dusky and there was some frothing at the mouth. She noticed that the woman's trousers were wet afterwards.

When the fit stopped the woman had appeared unconscious for a few minutes and then showed some response to being talked to but seemed confused and drowsy.

## Examination

She appears to be about 30 years old and in the third trimester of pregnancy. She is now conscious but still drowsy and her Glasgow Coma Scale is 9/15.

Her blood pressure is 140/98 mmHg and heart rate 104/min. Examination shows no obvious cardiac or chest abnormality, and on abdominal palpation there is no apparent tenderness. The uterus feels approximately 30-week size (midway between umbilicus and xiphisternum), and a fetus can be palpated, cephalic with 4/5 palpable. Reflexes are brisk and plantar reflexes are upgoing.

---

 **INVESTIGATIONS**

No investigation results are yet available for this patient when you see her.

---

## Questions

- What is your provisional diagnosis and how would you manage this woman in the first instance?
- The woman's husband arrives shortly and explains that she is a known epileptic who has grand mal seizures every few days, despite drug treatment. How should your management alter now?

# ANSWER 92

Any woman with a fit in the second half of pregnancy should be assumed to have eclampsia until proven otherwise. The risks of maternal or perinatal mortality are so great that it is better to treat the woman for eclampsia and prevent a further seizure than to spend time investigating and making a certain diagnosis while risking further fits. This case is therefore an obstetric emergency (despite the fact that the fit resolved spontaneously), and help should be summoned from the anaesthetist, senior midwife, senior obstetrician and paediatrician.

Magnesium sulphate should be given as an intravenous bolus of 4 g, followed by an infusion in normal saline of 1 g/h (increased if further fits occur).

Once this has been commenced, a urine sample should be acquired (with insertion of a Foley catheter to monitor urine output) for proteinuria. Fluid input should be restricted initially to 85 mL/h. Blood should be sent for full blood count, urea and electrolytes, urate, liver function tests, coagulation screen and group and save. She should be transferred to a high-dependency area of the labour ward with continuous electrocardiogram and cardiotocograph monitoring.

Once stable and further investigations have been made into her previous history, a decision can be made regarding delivery.

## Epilepsy diagnosis
The fact that the woman has epilepsy strongly suggests that this fit is caused by the epilepsy. However, the initial management was still correct as you will not be sure that the fit was due to this until the urinalysis has been confirmed to be normal and the blood pressure, initially high, has normalized, the reflexes returned to normal and the blood tests results are found to be normal.

Reflexes are commonly brisk, with upgoing plantar responses in the post-ictal phase.

This woman regained full consciousness after half an hour and the blood pressure was normal with negative urinalysis and normal blood results. The magnesium was thus discontinued and she was discharged with her husband, for neurological review within the next few days to discuss compliance and drug regime.

---

 **KEY POINTS**

- A woman who presents in the third trimester of pregnancy with a grand mal seizure should be treated as eclamptic until proven otherwise.

# CASE 93: BREATHLESSNESS IN PREGNANCY

## History

A 42-year-old woman is referred by her general practitioner with breathlessness for the past 3 days. She is 34 weeks pregnant in her third pregnancy. Prior to this she has had an emergency Caesarean section for abnormal cardiotocograph in labour, followed by a 7-week miscarriage.

In this pregnancy she was seen by the obstetric consultant to discuss plans for delivery, and is hoping for a vaginal delivery. Ultrasound scans and blood tests have been normal. Her booking blood pressure was 138/80 mmHg and has remained stable during the pregnancy.

She describes her shortness of breath starting while she was at work and slightly worsening since. She felt particularly breathless when she ran to catch a bus on her way home yesterday. She has some left-sided chest pain on breathing in. There is no cough or haemoptysis. She has had no previous episodes. She has not noticed any calf pain but has left leg swelling and some back pain.

## Examination

The body mass index is 28 kg/m$^2$. The woman does not look obviously unwell. Blood pressure is 127/78 mmHg and heart rate 98/min. Oxygen saturation is 96 per cent on air. On examination of the chest there is a systolic murmur and no added sounds. Chest expansion is normal but the woman reports pain on taking a deep breath. The chest is resonant to percussion and chest sounds are normal except for a pleural rub on the left. The left leg is generally swollen but no redness or tenderness is apparent.

---

### 🔍 INVESTIGATIONS

| | | Normal range for pregnancy |
|---|---|---|
| Haemoglobin | 12.0 g/dL | 11–14 g/dL |
| White cell count | 10.4 × 10$^9$/L | 6–16 × 10$^9$/L |
| Platelets | 302 × 10$^9$/L | 346 × 10$^9$/L |
| Arterial blood gas (on air): | | |
| paO$_2$ | 11.0 kPa | 12–14 kPa |
| paCO$_2$ | 5.3 kPa | 5–6 kPa |

D-dimer: positive

Electrocardiogram (ECG): sinus tachycardia 100/min, deep S wave in lead 1, Q wave in lead 3 and inverted T wave in lead 3

Chest X-ray: normal

Computerized tomography pulmonary angiogram (CTPA) is shown in Fig. 93.1.

---

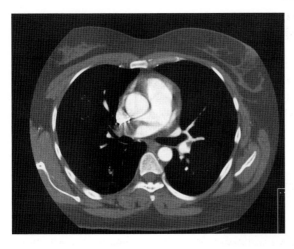

**Figure 93.1** Computed tomography pulmonary angiogram.

## Questions

- What is the diagnosis?
- What further imaging is required?
- How would you manage this woman in the immediate term, during delivery and postnatally?

## ANSWER 93

The diagnosis is of pulmonary embolism (PE). The shortness and breath and pleuritic chest pain are classic features, and the ECG and blood gas analysis support the diagnosis. D-dimer is commonly raised in pregnancy but also supports the diagnosis. The CTPA demonstrates a large filling defect within the right pulmonary artery and a smaller filling defect in the left segmental pulmonary artery, consistent with blood clots (pulmonary embolism). These findings are illustrated by the arrows in Fig. 93.2.

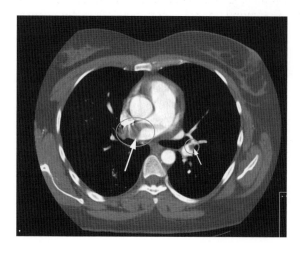

**Figure 93.2** CT pulmonary angiogram demonstrating a large filling defect in the right main pulmonary artery (large arrow) and smaller defect in a segmental branch of the left pulmonary artery (smaller arrow).

Venous thromboembolism (VTE) is the leading cause of direct deaths in the Confidential Enquiry into Maternal and Child Health, accounting for death in 1.2 per 100 000 maternities. Non-fatal VTE occurs in approximately 60 in 10 000 pregnancies, and there may be many more unrecognized cases. Pregnancy itself is a risk factor because of the hyper-oestrogenic state, the altered blood viscosity and obstruction to venous blood flow by the gravid uterus.

### Further imaging

There is no clinical evidence of calf ileofemoral deep vein thrombosis, but generalized leg swelling and back pain are suspicious of an ileofemoral thrombosis. If this is confirmed, which may require Doppler ultrasound or magnetic resonance imaging (or if she develops recurrent PE despite anticoagulation), then liaison with a vascular team should be considered regarding the possibility of insertion of a vena caval filter.

### Management

As with non-pregnant patients, anticoagulation is the mainstay of treatment. Warfarin is contraindicated in the first trimester of pregnancy but may safely be given from 12 to 36 weeks. However it can cause difficulties with excessive bleeding if it is not stopped early enough before delivery and it can be difficult to achieve stable international normalized ratio levels. Therefore low-molecular-weight heparin has become the treatment of choice in pregnancy as it is simple to administer, relatively easy to reverse in the emergency situation, does not require monitoring, and is safe.

At delivery the heparin should ideally be discontinued 12 h before delivery and recommenced immediately following delivery. Similarly an epidural or spinal anaesthetic should not be administered immediately after a heparin dose.

Postnatally some women change to warfarin, which is now known to be safe with breast-feeding, while others continue low-molecular-weight heparin.

A large proportion of VTE occurs postnatally, so anticoagulation should be continued for 6 weeks to 3 months in the puerperium.

Graduated elastic compression stocking should be worn from the time of diagnosis until at least 6 weeks following delivery, to reduce the risk of the post-thrombotic syndrome (chronic leg pain, swelling and ulceration).

Postnatal investigation for inherited (e.g. protein C or S deficiency) or acquired (e.g. anti-phospholipid syndrome) thrombophilia is appropriate, as is anticoagulation throughout any subsequent pregnancy.

---

 **KEY POINTS**

- Thromboembolic disease is common in pregnancy and one should have a high index of suspicion in making the diagnosis clinically.
- Anticoagulation should be given while waiting for confirmation of the diagnosis.

---

# CASE 94: BLOOD PRESSURE AND PREGNANCY

## History

A woman was admitted from the antenatal clinic two days ago at 38 weeks' gestation. She is 42 years old and this is her second pregnancy. Her first child was born by spontaneous vaginal delivery 13 years ago. She has subsequently remarried. Her booking blood pressure was 138/70 mmHg at 13 weeks. Her booking blood tests were unremarkable. At her 36 week midwife appointment 2 weeks ago, her blood pressure was 140/85 mmHg and the urinalysis was normal. The blood pressure was repeated 2 days later and was 140/82 mmHg. Two days ago she saw her midwife for a further appointment and her blood pressure was 148/101 mmHg. Urinalysis showed protein +.

She feels well in herself except for swollen legs. She denies any headache or blurring of vision.

## Examination

She has oedema to the mid calves and her fingers are swollen such that she cannot remove her rings. Abdominal palpation is non-tender and the symphysiofundal height is 39 cm. Reflexes are normal.

| INVESTIGATIONS | | |
|---|---|---|
| | | *Normal range for pregnancy* |
| Haemoglobin | 12.4 g/dL | 11–14 g/dL |
| White cell count | 8 × 10⁹/L | 6–16 × 10⁹/L |
| Packed cell volume | 34% | 31–38% |
| Platelets | 210 × 10⁹/L | 150–400 × 10⁹/L |
| Sodium | 137 mmol/L | 130–140 mmol/L |
| Potassium | 3.9 mmol/L | 3.3–4.1 mmol/L |
| Urea | 2.5 mmol/L | 2.4–4.3 mmol/L |
| Creatinine | 80 μmol/L | 34–82 μmol/L |
| Alanine transaminase | 37 IU/L | 6–32 IU/L |
| Alkaline phosphatase | 98 IU/L | 30–300 IU/L |
| Bilirubin | 10 μmol/L | (3–14 micromol/L) |
| Gamma glutamyl transaminase | 32 IU/L | 5–43 IU/L |
| Urate | 43 mmol/L | (0.14–0.38 mmol/L) |

24-h urinary protein collection: volume 1.8 L; total protein 2.16 g; protein per litre 1.2 g

## Questions

- How would you interpret the investigations?
- What further investigations are needed and how should she be managed?

# ANSWER 94

## Results interpretation

The haemoglobin and packed cell volume suggest mild haemoconcentration. The platelet count is normal for pregnancy, though low for a non-pregnant person. Electrolytes are within the normal range but the creatinine is higher than normal for pregnancy. Alkaline phosphatase is always raised in pregnancy due to its production by the placenta. However the alanine transaminase is abnormal.

A normal urate value correlates with gestational age (the urate level should not be more than the number of weeks gestation) and therefore the level of 43 mmol/L is high. Finally, the 24-h urinary protein measurement, performed to quantify the degree of proteinuria, has shown a significantly raised result.

This woman thus has pregnancy-induced hypertension (PIH) with proteinuria, abnormal liver function and raised serum creatinine and urate. This is known as pre-eclampsia. The condition commonly occurs in asymptomatic women and the severity of symptoms often does not correlate with the disease severity.

No further maternal investigations are needed but fetal wellbeing needs to be assessed by cardiotocograph and ultrasound assessment for fetal growth and liquor volume in view of the association between pre-eclampsia and intrauterine growth restriction.

Induction of labour as soon as possible is indicated, as the fetus is beyond 37 weeks and delay might increase the likelihood of fulminating pre-eclampsia in the mother or fetal compromise, including placental abruption. There is no indication for Caesarean section unless induction is unsuccessful or fetal compromise occurs before or during labour. Close monitoring of blood pressure is imperative during and after labour, as many eclamptic fits occur postnatally.

In this case the woman agreed to induction of labour and started contracting after the first dose of intravaginal prostaglandin gel. The labour progressed rapidly with subsequent normal delivery. However the blood pressure increased in labour to 155/110 mmHg. An epidural was sited to help reduce the blood pressure. Blood pressure increased further and a hydralazine infusion was required.

She remained in hospital for 5 days postpartum for blood pressure monitoring, during which time her blood results returned to normal. Postnatally she was converted to oral labetalol for 6 weeks, after which blood pressure was normal, and treatment discontinued.

---

 KEY POINTS

- Pre-eclampsia is common and is associated with significant maternal morbidity and mortality.
- Proteinuria should be quantified with analysis of a 24-h urine collection.

# CASE 95: LABOUR

## History

A 22-year-old woman is admitted to the labour ward for induction of labour at 39 weeks' gestation. This is her first ongoing pregnancy, having had a first-trimester miscarriage 13 months previously. She booked at 9 weeks and had normal booking blood tests, and 11–14-week scan and 21-week anomaly scan did not show any obvious fetal abnormality. Blood pressure and urinalysis have always been normal.

At her 32 week midwife appointment she reported feeling very uncomfortable abdominally, and the midwife measured the symphysiofundal height to be 36 cm. A further ultrasound scan was therefore requested whish showed normal fetal growth but increased liquor volume. She had been reviewed in the antenatal clinic and was tested for gestational diabetes with glucose tolerance test but this was normal. Subsequent examinations had again confirmed an increased symphysiofundal height, and further ultrasound scan at 36 weeks again showed normal growth, no fetal abnormality and markedly increased liquor volume. The fetal movements had always been normal.

A decision had been made for induction of labour at 40 weeks because the woman had become so uncomfortable and breathless.

On palpation the fetus was cephalic with the head 4/5 palpable abdominally. Cardiotocograph (CTG) was reassuring; 2 mg of prostaglandin gel had been inserted into the posterior fornix of the vagina and CTG monitoring continued for a further 20 min.

The woman then mobilized and contractions started within an hour. She requested an epidural for analgesia and while this was being prepared CTG monitoring was commenced. At this stage, spontaneous rupture of membranes occurred with a very large volume of clear liquor soaking the bed sheets.

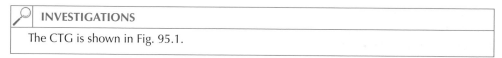

INVESTIGATIONS

The CTG is shown in Fig. 95.1.

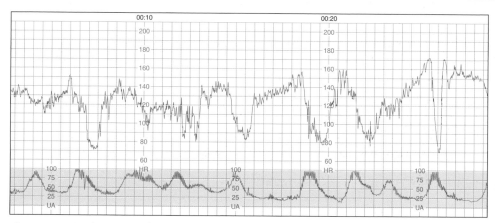

**Figure 95.1** Cardiotocograph.

## Questions
- Describe the CTG
- What is the likely diagnosis?
- How would you confirm the diagnosis and manage this situation?

# ANSWER 95

The CTG shows deep variable decelerations. The sudden CTG deterioration after rupture of membranes in a woman with polyhydramnios suggests the likelihood of prolapse of the cord. Other possible diagnoses are placental abruption or fetal head compression from precipitate labour. The diagnosis is easily confirmed with vaginal examination. A loop of umbilical cord will be palpated in the vagina and will be pulsatile.

| ! | Risk factors for cord prolapse |
|---|---|
| | • Polyhydramnios<br>• Preterm delivery<br>• Malpresentation<br>• Unstable presentation<br>• Multiple pregnancy |

This is an obstetric emergency and the emergency bell should be activated with the senior midwife, theatre team, senior obstetrician, paediatrician and anaesthetist summoned immediately.

The important management steps are:

- the examiner should not remove their fingers from the vagina and should attempt to elevate the fetal head above the cord and minimize contact with the cord to prevent spasm
- the woman should be rotated into the 'all-fours position' (head lower than buttocks), which will facilitate relieving the weight of the baby and abdomen from the prolapsed cord
- she should be transferred to theatre immediately for Caesarean section
- intravenous access should be obtained, and a general anaesthetic administered, using a rapid sequence induction with cricoid pressure
- the examiner should only remove their fingers from the presenting part in the vagina when the uterus has been opened and the baby is being delivered.

| 🔍 | KEY POINTS |
|---|---|
| | • Cord prolapse should be suspected in cases of fetal heart abnormality occurring after rupture of membranes.<br>• It is an obstetric emergency and necessitates immediate Caesarean section.<br>• Attempts should be made to minimize pressure on the cord pending delivery. |

## CASE 96: NEONATAL CARE

### History

A 19-year-old woman is in spontaneous labour at 37 weeks 2 days' gestation. At 4 cm cervical dilatation there is thick meconium liquor and a fetal heart deceleration to 70/min is heard lasting for 2 min. The woman is immediately placed on the continuous cardiotogograph (CTG), which confirms regular deep late decelerations.

A decision is made to deliver the baby by immediate Caesarean section under general anaesthetic. The baby is delivered within 20 min.

---

**INVESTIGATIONS**

*Apgar score at 1 min*:

Heart rate: <100/min: 1

Respiratory effort: absent: 0

Muscle tone: some flexion: 1

Reflex grimace: 1

Colour pale/blue: 0

Total Apgar score: 3

*Umbilical cord blood samples*:

Arterial blood gas: pH 7.01; base excess −12.8 mmol/L

Venous blood gas: pH 7.12; base excess −11.5 mmol/L

---

### Questions

- How do you interpret the Apgar and cord blood results?
- What action would you take in these circumstances?

# ANSWER 96

The Apgar score is a simple scoring system to record the initial assessment of neonates in the first few minutes after delivery. For each variable a score of 0, 1 or 2 may be allocated (see Table 96.1).

Table 96.1 **Apgar scores**

| | Score | | |
|---|---|---|---|
| | **0** | **1** | **2** |
| Heart rate | Absent | <100/min | >100/min |
| Respiratory effort | Absent | Gasp/shallow breaths | Normal/crying |
| Muscle tone | Limp | Some flexion | Flexion |
| Reflex | None | Grimace | Cough/cry |
| Colour | Pale/blue | Blue extremities | Pink |

In this case the baby is clearly showing no respiratory effort and is bradycardic at birth. The arterial cord blood shows an acidosis.

## Management

Most babies, even with low Apgar scores respond to initial resuscitation measures:

- immediately dry the baby with warm towels, replacing any wet towels with dry ones
- warm by wrapping in a warm dry towel and placing under the heated rescuscitaire
- stimulate by rubbing (during drying)
- if no immediate respiratory effort is made then proceed to 5 inflationary breaths with oxygen via a self-limiting pressure bag and appropriately sized face mask (most babies will respond and immediately increase their heart rate and begin to make some respiratory effort)
- recheck the respiration and heart rate. If they have not recovered, clear the airway with gentle suction (this baby has been exposed to thick meconium which may have been inhaled and be causing a mechanical obstruction)
- if the heart rate is above 60/min, continue ventilation with bag and mask until heart rate increases to above 100/min
- if the heart rate is below 60/min begin chest compressions, continue bag and mask ventilation and check that the neonatal resuscitation team has been called.

This baby recovered its heart rate and respiratory effort with the first three measures but continued to display 'grunting' respiratory effort, and 3 h later deteriorated and needed ventilation. A diagnosis of meconium aspiration and pneumonitis was made and antibiotics and supportive measures were initiated with final extubation after 7 days and discharge home 5 days later.

---

 **KEY POINTS**

- All health professionals delivering babies must be able to perform basic neonatal resuscitation.
- The majority of babies with low Apgar score at delivery respond to initial drying and warming.

# FAMILY PLANNING AND SEXUAL HEALTH

## CASE 97: UNPROTECTED INTERCOURSE

### History
A 21-year-old woman presents because she has had unprotected intercourse and is worried about pregnancy. She has been on holiday and met a man with whom she had unprotected intercourse 36 h ago, and also 4 days before that.

Her last menstrual period started 13 days ago and she bleeds for 4 days every 27 days. She has had no other episodes of intercourse since her last period. She is generally healthy but has a history of epilepsy for which she takes carbamazepine. She has no other significant medical history.

### Examination
Abdominal examination is unremarkable and internal examination is not indicated.

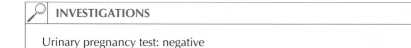

| INVESTIGATIONS |
| --- |
| Urinary pregnancy test: negative |

### Questions
• What options are available to this woman and how should she be managed?

# ANSWER 97

Two forms of emergency contraception are generally available:

- emergency intrauterine contraceptive device (IUCD)
- hormonal emergency contraception (levonorgestrel).

Hormonal emergency contraception involves 1.5 mg levonorgestrel, taken as soon as possible after intercourse (preferably within 12 h). It is effective up to 72 h and can be given safely up to 5 days (unlicensed), but the earlier it is taken, the more effective it is. In this case the woman has had intercourse more than 72 h ago and therefore this method should be assumed to be ineffective. She is also taking an enzyme-inducing drug and should therefore be advised, if she were suitable to use this method, to take a higher dose of levonorgestrel (3 mg).

---

**!** **Advice after emergency hormonal contraception**

- Nausea is a common side-effect and women can be given prophylactic domperidone. If vomiting occurs, domperidone and a second levonorgestrel dose should be given as soon as possible.
- A barrier method of contraception needs to be used until the next period.
- The next period may be early or late, but if it is very late or very unusual she should take a pregnancy test.
- She needs to return promptly if lower abdominal pain occurs, to rule out an ectopic pregnancy.

---

## Emergency intrauterine contraceptive device

This woman should be advised to have an emergency IUCD inserted, and although she has never been pregnant this is unlikely to be a problem as IUCDs can generally be inserted under local anaesthetic, even in nulliparous women.

It can be inserted up to 120 h (5 days) after unprotected intercourse. If intercourse has occurred more than 5 days previously, the intrauterine device can still be inserted up to 5 days after the earliest likely calculated ovulation. In this case the earliest likely ovulation is today (taking account of her 27-day cycle).

The IUCD is also more effective than the hormonal emergency contraception whenever used. Insertion needs to be covered by antibacterial prophylaxis to prevent pelvic inflammatory disease.

A pregnancy test should always be taken before any emergency contraception, whatever the menstrual history. Women should also be advised to consider sexually transmitted infection testing after unprotected intercourse with a new partner, and should be encouraged to use a reliable regular method of contraception.

---

 **KEY POINTS**

- The emergency IUCD is more effective than emergency hormonal contraception and can be used up to 5 days after the earliest calculated ovulation date, even if this is more than 5 days after unprotected intercourse.

---

## CASE 98: VAGINAL DISCHARGE

### History

A 19-year-old woman presents with a vaginal discharge. She is currently 9 weeks pregnant in her first pregnancy. The discharge started about 3 weeks ago and is non-itchy and creamy in colour. It is not profuse but she feels it has a strong odour and is embarrassed about it. There is no bleeding or abdominal pain. She has had two or three previous similar episodes before the pregnancy that resolved spontaneously.

She has been with her partner for 3 years and neither of them have had any other sexual partners. They have always used condoms until 3 months ago. She has never had a cervical smear test.

### Examination

The external genitalia appear normal. On speculum examination a small amount of smooth grey discharge is seen coating the vagina walls. There is a small cervical ectropion that is not bleeding.

### Questions
- What is the likely diagnosis and the differential diagnosis?
- How would you further investigate and manage this patient?
- If your diagnosis is confirmed, what are the implications for the pregnancy?

# ANSWER 98

The history suggests that the woman is not at risk of a sexually transmitted infection as a cause for her discharge (although this can never be ruled out entirely as the reported sexual history can be inaccurate). She has an ectropion, which can cause a clear discharge. A non-offensive, non-itchy discharge is normal in pregnancy.

The salient feature in this case is that the discharge has an offensive odour. Offensive odour is usually due to either trichomonas or bacterial vaginosis (BV). Trichomonas causes a profuse, sometimes frothy discharge with cervicitis, whereas BV causes a smooth, mild discharge, if any discharge at all.

---

**!  Differential diagnosis of vaginal discharge**

- Infective
  - sexually transmitted
    - trichomonas
    - chlamydia
    - gonorrhoea
  - non-sexually transmitted
    - candida
    - bacterial vaginosis
- Physiological
  - pregnancy
  - ovulation
- Cervical ectropion

---

## Further investigation

The woman should have swabs taken for sexually transmitted infection as well as BV and candida.

A diagnosis of BV can be made, finding a typical thin grey discharge with a fishy odour and a vaginal pH of 6–7. More formal criteria for diagnosis are the Amsel (discharge, clue cells on microscopy, high pH and fishy odour with potassium hydroxide) or Hay/Ison criteria (relative lactobacilli to anaerobe proportions on Gram-stained vaginal smear). Microbiological culture is not helpful as many of the anaerobes associated with BV are also found as commensals.

## Management

Spontaneous onset and remission is typical with BV, and 50 per cent of women are asymptomatic. General advice should be given for avoiding BV including avoidance of vaginal douching, shower gel, and antiseptic agents or shampoo in the bath, as these interfere with the normal flora (lactobacilli) and allow an increase in BV organisms.

Specific treatment is with metronidazole for 5–7 days.

## BV and pregnancy

Late miscarriage, preterm birth, preterm premature rupture of membranes, and postpartum endometritis have all been associated with BV, and so any pregnant woman with BV should be treated with metronidazole. In contrast, non-pregnant women only require treatment if symptomatic.

**KEY POINTS**

- BV is a common cause of discharge and is the most likely diagnosis in a woman complaining of an offensive or 'fishy' odour, but a full sexually transmitted infection screen is usually indicated to rule out other co-existing infection.
- Treatment with metronidazole is indicated in all affected pregnant women, but in non-pregnant women it is only indicated for those with symptoms.

## CASE 99: TEENAGE CONTRACEPTION

### History

A 14-year-old girl attends a family planning clinic wanting to start 'the pill'. She has been with her boyfriend for 8 months. They both agreed that they wanted to start a sexual relationship and have already had intercourse on two occasions where they did not use contraception. She had never been sexually active before. Her periods started 3 years ago and were initially irregular but she now reports a regular 27-day cycle. She has never had any gynaecological or other medical problems.

She reports that she is happy at school and she is one of three children, with a brother of 21 and sister of 19 years. She lives with her parents in a house locally. She has attended the clinic with a female school friend.

### Examination

There are no examination or investigations findings.

### Questions

- What issues are important in determining how this situation should be managed?
- How would you further investigate, advise and manage this girl?

# ANSWER 99

Prescribing of contraception to girls under the legal age of consent (16 years) is guided by the Fraser Rules, which arose from the case of Gillick seeking to stop a doctor from providing contraceptive advice to her daughter without consulting the parents.

The law allows contraception to be provided as long as the following criteria are met:

- the girl should be encouraged to discuss her sexual activity with a parent or another responsible adult
- she should consent to intercourse
- she should understand the implications of having sexual intercourse and the contraceptive method chosen
- it is anticipated that she will have sex whether or not contraception is provided and is therefore at potentially higher physical and psychological harm from an inadvertent pregnancy.

In this case it is clear that the girl will continue to have sex with or without contraception as she has already done so, and therefore it is in her best interests to prevent pregnancy. She should be encouraged to discuss the issue with a parent, or failing this perhaps her older sister or brother.

The age of her boyfriend should be explored – if he is of a similar age then consent is probably valid. However if there is a significant age discrepancy, for example he was over 20 years, then issues of child protection should be considered and the case should be discussed in the first instance with a social worker.

## Investigation and advice

A urinary pregnancy test should be performed prior to any hormonal contraception, as she has already had unprotected intercourse.

She should be advised about the different methods of contraception, particularly how to use them and the importance of compliance. The availability of emergency contraception should be explained.

She is at risk of sexually transmitted infections, and barrier contraception should be advised even if she is using the contraceptive pill as her main pregnancy-prevention strategy.

Whichever option is chosen, the girl should be supported such that she is happy to come back for further review and to check correct usage of the preferred method. Explanation of confidentiality rules will also aid her confidence in your advice.

---

 **KEY POINTS**

- Contraception may be provided to girls under the age of 16 years without parental consent subject to the guidance in the Fraser rules.
- Sexually transmitted infections and education about emergency contraception are an integral part of such consultations.

# CASE 100: INTERMENSTRUAL BLEEDING

## History

A 21-year-old student presents with vaginal bleeding between her periods. It first occurred 2 months ago and she has had several recurrences. It is usually light and generally lasts from 1 to 3 days.

She has been on the combined oral contraceptive pill (COCP) for 18 months and has regular periods, lasting for 3 days every 28 days. The periods are not heavy or painful. She has not noticed any other discharge. She has not had any bowel or urinary symptoms.

She first had sexual intercourse at the age of 17 years and has been with her current boyfriend for 4 months. There is no pain on intercourse and no postcoital bleeding.

She was seen once before in the gynaecology clinic for pelvic pain and was noted to have a simple ovarian cyst, which subsequently resolved spontaneously. She has no other significant medical history of note. The general practitioner had arranged an ultrasound assessment prior to referral.

## Examination

She is slim and looks well. The abdomen is not distended and is non-tender. The external genitalia are normal and on speculum examination a slight blood-stained discharge is noted coming from the cervical os. There is a cervical ectropion which is not bleeding.

Bimanual examination reveals an aneteverted normal size mobile uterus. There is no cervical excitation or adnexal tenderness.

---

 **INVESTIGATIONS**

*Transvaginal ultrasound examination*:

The uterus is normal size and anteverted. The endometrium measures 7 mm in anteroposterior diameter and is regular along its entire length.

Both ovaries appear of normal size and morphology.

There is no free peritoneal fluid.

*Urinary pregnancy test*: negative.

---

## Questions
- What is the differential diagnosis?
- How would you further investigate and manage this woman?

## ANSWER 100

The symptom of bleeding between the pill-free interval in a woman taking the combined oral contraceptive pill is known as breakthrough bleeding. It can have many causes and a good history should include, in addition to the history given:

- has she been missing any pills?
- has she taken any other medication which might interefere with the COCP (e.g. antibiotics, enzyme inducers)?
- has she had any intercurrent illnesses causing diarrhoea or vomiting?
- has she ever had any sexually transmitted infections, or been investigated for this?
- how many sexual partners has she had in the last 3 months?
- has she recently changed the COCP that she uses?

The differential diagnosis in a woman with breakthrough bleeding is

- COCP-related causes
  - poor compliance
  - intercurrent infection causing poor pill absorption
  - drug interactions, reducing the COCP efficacy
  - inadequate oestrogen component for that woman
  - pregnancy
- unrelated causes
  - cervical ectropion
  - sexually transmitted infection – chlamydia, gonorrhoea, trichomonas
  - candidal vaginitis
  - cervical or endometrial polyp
  - bleeding disorder (rare).

The woman should have the following swabs taken:

- endocervical – for chlamydia
- high vaginal – for trichomonas or candida
- endocervical – for gonorrhoea.

(Bacterial vaginosis is another vaginal infection but does not cause bleeding.)

Chlamydia is an increasingly common infection, especially in women aged 18–24 years. It is commonly asymptomatic or may present with minimal symptoms as in this case. It should be tested for with endocervical swab, though urine testing and low vaginal swab testing are also possible. If confirmed, the woman should be treated with doxyxcline or azithromycin and advised that her partner(s) should also be tested and treated at a genitourinary medicine clinic before they resume intercourse.

If the swabs are negative and no other cause can be identified for the breakthrough bleeding, then the woman should be changed to an alternative contraceptive pill. There is no clear solution to suit all women, but possibilities are a phasic pill, an alternative progestogen (such as a 'third-generation' progestogen) or a pill containing a higher dose of oestrogen (50 µg rather than 30 µg).

**KEY POINTS**

- Breakthrough bleeding with the combined oral contraceptive pill can have many causes.
- Chlamydia infection is often asymptomatic or presents with vague symptoms such as irregular bleeding.
- Compliance with medication, contact tracing and avoidance of sexual intercourse until completion of treatment by both partners is essential in the management of chlamydia infection.

# INDEX

References are by case number with relevant page numbers following in brackets. References with a page range e.g. 25(68–70) indicate that although the subject may be mentioned only on one page, it concerns the whole case.